Advance Praise for *Parenting Your Parents*:

"A practical, no-nonsense book filled with honest emotion and valuable planning tools and references."

Susan Donaldson, CEO
Ontario Association of Community Care Access Centres

"Parentcare for both the experienced and uninitiated. Frank, compassionate, and intimate, Mindszenthy and Gordon tell it like it is."

Caroline Tapp-McDougall, Publisher
Solutions Magazine

"A wonderfully readable, useful guide and comprehensive resource for the boomer generation as they struggle with the challenges of caring for their aging parents. Readers will recognize themselves and their parents in the many vignettes on which this book is based."

Howard Bergman, MD
The Dr. Joseph Kaufmann Chair in Geriatric Medicine
Professor and Director of Geriatric Medicine, McGill University

"Bart Mindszenthy and Dr. Michael Gordon will earn the thanks of innumerable readers for their informative case histories and sage advice about family tensions, social issues, and medical challenges that arise as our parents age."

David Naylor, MD DPhil FRCPC
Dean, Faculty of Medicine, University of Toronto

"A well-written, excellent resource book. Every family should have a copy."

Nadine Henningsen, Executive Director
Canadian Home Care Association

"This book provides compassionate and helpful advice for the difficult end-of-life issues that emerge as we care for those we love."

Julie White, CEO
Canadian Cancer Society/National Cancer Institute of Canada

PARENTING YOUR PARENTS

Support Strategies for Meeting the Challenge of Aging in the Family

Bart Mindszenthy and Michael Gordon, MD

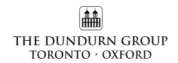

THE DUNDURN GROUP
TORONTO · OXFORD

Copy-editor: Ruth Wilson
Designer: Jennifer Scott
Printer: Transcontinental

National Library of Canada Cataloguing in Publication Data

Mindszenthy, Bart J., 1946-
    Parenting your parents : support strategies for meeting the challenge of aging in the family

Includes bibliographical references.
ISBN 1-55002-380-2

1. Aging parents--Care. 2. Parent and adult child. I. Gordon, Michael, 1941- II. Title.

HQ1063.6.M55 2002   306.874   C2002-901073-X

1   2   3   4   5   06   05   04   03   02

   Canada

THE CANADA COUNCIL | LE CONSEIL DES ARTS
FOR THE ARTS | DU CANADA
SINCE 1957 | DEPUIS 1957

ONTARIO ARTS COUNCIL
CONSEIL DES ARTS DE L'ONTARIO

We acknowledge the support of the **Canada Council for the Arts** and the **Ontario Arts Council** for our publishing program. We also acknowledge the financial support of the **Government of Canada** through the **Book Publishing Industry Development Program** and **The Association for the Export of Canadian Books**, and the **Government of Ontario** through the **Ontario Book Publishers Tax Credit** program.

Care has been taken to trace the ownership of copyright material used in this book. The author and the publisher welcome any information enabling them to rectify any references or credit in subsequent editions.

J. Kirk Howard, President

Printed and bound in Canada.⊛
Printed on recycled paper.
www.dundurn.com

Dundurn Press
8 Market Street
Suite 200
Toronto, Ontario, Canada
M5E 1M6

Dundurn Press
73 Lime Walk
Headington, Oxford,
England
OX3 7AD

Dundurn Press
2250 Military Road
Tonawanda NY
U.S.A. 14150

To our parents,
whose lifelong legacy of love and caring
serve to guide and inspire us.

TABLE OF CONTENTS

Acknowledgements

A SPECIAL THANK YOU TO THOSE who gave us encouragement and support most every day throughout the process of writing this book: Michael's wife, Gilda Berger, and sister, Diane Gordon; Bart's partner, Gail Roberts, and ever-inquiring and interested father, Bart Sr.

A warm thank you to Dr. Robert Horvath, who arranged for us to meet and discover that we, indeed, could work very together.

Much appreciation also to Caroline Tapp-McDougall, publisher of *Solutions* magazine and the Baycrest Centre for Geriatric Care for sharing research into support resources available nationally. From that foundation, many hours were spent updating and expanding the directory, with special help from Glenn Hildebrand in Winnipeg, who worked so hard to refine it further; Gerard Godbout in Hull, Que.; Rod Stanely in Summerside, PEI; Leanne Tait in Yellowknife, NWT; Joel Wiener, Health Canada's Regional Director for Ontario and his staff; and all the nice people in provincial ministries and with various associations who were so kind with their time.

Also many thanks to Mona Munro and Renne Climens of the Department of Social Work at the Baycrst Centre for Geriatric Care for their input and comments.

Finally, we are delighted with Dundurn Press' keen interest in this book, starting with Tony Hawke's deep conviction that the time was right and ripe for *Parenting Your Parents*; and Beth Bruder, who made the original connection because she knew first hand of the need; and, Barry Jowett, our superb editorial coordinator who did a magnificent job keeping us on track.

And, to all of you who told us stories of your own personal experiences...thank you for sharing openly your own personal and family challenges.

FOREWORD

by
Sandie Rinaldo

WHO CAN'T HELP BUT LEARN FROM BORIS, Bob, Ivan and Sophie? Ivan and Sophie are elderly parents who've been encouraged by their well-intentioned sons, Boris and Bob, to leave their home in Red Deer and move to Montreal to be near them. What begins as a tender reunion sours quickly as family pressures intermingle with filial responsibilities. Wives are unhappy. Grandchildren disinterested. And sadly, Ivan and Sophie feel misplaced and long to return to the old way of life.

Theirs is but one of dozens of anecdotes the authors have collected in a storytelling anthology that explores an important and timely topic.

You might recognize yourself in Boris and Bob; or in Sylvia, whose mother Lee Ann is plagued by ill health; or Edna Delaney's four children, whose sibling rivalry and mutual distrust have placed enormous stress on Edna's well-being; or Dorothy Miller, who's family must cope with her advancing dementia.

From surviving a stroke to reigning in the rebellious grandmother, from angst to xenophobia, the authors let the many stories carry the book. They chart the challenge, and offer advice.

Perhaps that's what makes this book so unique. It's not a sophisticated treatise laced with medical lingo, but rather the kind of read that's reminiscent of a descriptive, fictional novel. And yet, the stories and characters in *Parenting Your Parents* are real.

Two real gems round out the book: a Personal Parenting Planner — which serves as a status check, a fact-gathering repository, and an action planner; and a Resource Directory — a who-to-call lifeline.

As the sandwich generation, we live in the new reality, where isolation is a factor, and where families and neighbourhood roles are changing. We have much to learn from the shared experiences of others.

Boris and Bob taught me that sometimes it's wiser to help parents live their lives instead of pushing an agenda because you think it might be better for them. My dad will thank them for my new-found wisdom. He thrives on independence and as long as he is healthy and of good mind, he should continue to live life to the fullest.

Consider this book a valuable resource.

Sandie Rinaldo
February 2002

Preface

Parenting Your Parents —
Stepping Into the Unkown

THEY'RE NOW VERY OLD AND FRAIL: my parents. I'm told by so many that I'm fortunate to still have them. The people who tell me this lost their own parents when they were still relatively young—in their late sixties and early seventies.

As we start to work on this book, my mother is 86 years old, and my father is getting close to 96. They're fragile. They're proud. They're fiercely determined. They're more the exception than the rule, given their ages.

They still live in their North York home, and every day they get up, wash, dress, make their beds, and eat their breakfast. They work very hard at making their lives as normal as they can, and it's somewhat like watching a movie in slow motion for most of us, since they just simply move more slowly and everything takes longer.

I'm proud of them. I'm afraid for them. I'm confused about my role, my obligation. I know we're marking time. I can see it every time I'm with them. Their strength and determination are fading and being replaced by sheer will and a kind of day-to-day disciplined routine that keeps them going.

They're very social, but very private. They don't want people they don't know to come and help them. It's almost like some kind of threat. So they depend on me — and on a young married woman who comes three or four times a week to help them bathe, clean, cook, and run errands. Without her being there, I really don't know what I'd do or how I'd cope with where we are in the end game of their lives.

And that's precisely where we are. The end game. They know it. I know it. We don't talk about it too much, but that's the reality we elect to ignore as often and for as long as we can.

My parents are unique and amazing. But so are all parents. There are no two sets alike, anywhere, ever. They're what we get at birth. They're the link to the past and our passports to the future. Most parents do the best they can, no matter what we think or feel in the course of life. They weren't "trained" in parenthood, so they made up rules and procedures as they went along. Or they read Dr. Spock and followed the strict guidelines that long since have been denounced.

No matter which course they took, our parents struggled and strove to do what they thought was best for us in preparing us for the future. They imparted in us lifelong values and beliefs we may not realize or, perhaps, too seldom challenge. They planted in us views and traits we practise and uphold without always understanding. They were, and often still are, more influential in our lives than we can ever acknowledge or even comprehend.

Parents are special. We love to love them, and we sometimes try to hate them. There are times we see them as an intrusive burden, and at times we long to cut the chains that bind us. But seldom, if ever, can we walk away from them. Or even want to.

Our parents are simply there—with us, for us. They are an integral part of our world — in our minds, in our lives, sometimes in the way. Never out of the way, until they die. And when they do, there is an immense emotional outflow of fear, love, loss, anger, and confusion. For these are the people who so influenced who and what we are today, and more often than not, we don't even realize the impact they have until they're gone.

We who wrote this book, and everyone reading it, are trapped by the indisputable fact that the old rules and structures that drove the family compact are virtually non-existent. Just consider:

Our parents, most of whom were born in the first third of the 20th century, were reared with values and family and social expectations that have radically changed in the past 20 years. The difference between their paradigm and ours is probably greater than any other back-to-back generations.

Advances in medicine and major improvements in our quality of life mean people are living longer than ever—and our parents are the first generation to truly benefit —but not without paying a price.

We baby boomers and our children are more mobile than any generation before. Many of us change where we live and work more often than ever. For many, that means there is the added dimension of distance between our parents and us.

The two-income family is commonplace, putting added pressure on us to spend time helping our own children, who are more often returning to the family nest at some point in their lives for a period of time. So there is less time to spend supporting parents in need than there was in the 1950s and 1960s, when the wife and mother of a family had a traditional role as homemaker and supporter that was clear and socially acceptable at the time.

There is a relatively new phenomenon of "multi-parent children": those whose parents have divorced and remarried or are living in common-law relationships. New challenges centre around emotions, loyalties, and priorities in considering how to best apply attention and energy in supporting not two, but possibly three or four "parents."

The major changes that governments have introduced in the past decade to cut costs and taxes have resulted in a strain on services for the aging offered by the not-for-profit sector.

Where does all this leave you and me? Usually, between a rock and a hard place that is stifling, intimidating, and frightening.

But all of us who have aging parents want to help them. The challenge is helping them without becoming captives in the process: captives to parent care and parent over-dependency. It's a tough balancing act, with no set rules and myriad but confusing support mechanisms. We're in uncharted waters, and the water is deep and cold and treacherous.

So back to my parents and how I came to know them.

Late on the evening of June 12, 1946, a midwife nudged and eased me from my mother's warm, safe womb into the confusing, devastated, hurtful, hateful, hungry world of post-World War II Europe.

And so I was born, the only child of my parents. Hungarian by birth, but a citizen of a new world. For the first few years of my life, we lived hand-to-mouth as refugees in Bavaria. We were "DPs"—displaced persons: people who had lost their homeland, their homes, and all their possessions. People who were trying to find a new life because the war had taken everything from them. Then, in the summer of 1949, we were sponsored to come to America, the land of dreams and hope. We arrived in Detroit with one suitcase. My father weighed all of 99 pounds, and my mother was ill. But we managed to cross the Atlantic on an old 11,000-ton troop carrier crammed with others seeking a new life in a new world.

There was nothing glamorous about my early years. My parents worked hard at learning English and their jobs, and they tried as best they could to give me all that a little kid might expect. Except in my case, for the first number of years, what I got was used clothing and hand-me-down toys.

I remember a lot of things that aren't terribly relevant. What is relevant is that they tried so hard to bring joy and direction to my world, and they gave it with as much love and affection as they knew how.

Now, more than half a century later, we're into role reversal. I am the "parent," and they are the ones who need care, attention, support, and loving. But now we're in another country—Canada, where I came in 1969, and where my parents followed after retirement in 1973.

My father is now legally blind; his bodily functions are working relatively well considering his age, but everything in his day-to-day world is happening in slow motion. My mother's memory is faltering, mainly because of the sleeping pills to which she's become addicted.

I live 12 kilometres away from them — not a big distance except during rush hours and snowstorms. Every other day, I make it a point to see them, to spend some time talking with them, and doing things for them.

As I look back on where we've been and where we are, what I sense and feel is that through all the turmoil and upheaval of the past five-plus decades, my parents did the best they could to protect and help me, to make my little world safe and secure. And as I listen and learn from others, I hear that they, too, for the most part, remember parents who did the best they could to protect and help them, wherever they were at the time. And that's maybe the single most important thing we all have in common: parents who did the best they could for us.

Now, we've got to return the favour. We've got to help them as they become more and more helpless, just like they helped us when we were helpless. Nice and noble to say, but in today's world, it's very hard to do. If we're honest with ourselves, we know that while we love our parents, this is not something we want to be doing. And we're unsure because most of us don't quite know how to approach being caregivers in the best way possible.

So the bottom line question is this: Do we have the will, the energy, the power, the resources, and the commitment to do it? Or, put another way, do we have a moral choice?

Yes, we're ever thoughtful about our careers. Yes, we want to be secure financially. Yes, we want our kids to forge their own lives while we help them the best we can. And yes, we live in a confusing, uncertain, ever-changing world. But aside from all that, we have parents who are aging and in various conditions of decay (because what else can we call it if we're facing the cold facts?) and fully cognizant that we're all marking time.

So here we are, in our forties and fifties with a growing set of unwanted responsibilities that we can face and address, or we can ignore. And it all comes down to choices. Hard choices. Confusing and challenging choices. And that's what this book is all about.

Whether or not we agree with what our parents did in the past or what they're doing now, they are our parents. Were it not for them, we wouldn't be. But we are. And because we are, we must care for them in their times of need.

Most of us say we love our parents, and most of us really do. All we need to remind ourselves of that sacred emotion is to think back on the myriad good memories stored deep in our minds. Or to think about those silly occasions when we did truly dumb things and our parents got us through them with a good laugh and some good advice. Or to think about how we all laughed and hugged and celebrated special events and achievements. And the moments when we were afraid and they gave us comfort and confidence. And to remember how they worried about us, and tried to give us advice we often ignored, and how they stood by us through our personal trials and tribulations as we crossed the invisible boundary between youth and adulthood.

Parenting Your Parents is about you. About what you will want and need to think through as you embark on a tumultuous journey of caring about and for your aging parents. Or about what you need to consider right now, because you haven't planned or prepared for the onslaught of challenges that surely will bear down on you with an intensity and weight you simply won't have anticipated.

Parenting Your Parents looks at what people just like you are facing and examines how everyone is coping. And it's rich with the thoughts, ideas, and advice of one of Canada's pre-eminent geriatric health care professionals who provides counsel and support every year to hundreds of elderly people in need of expert insight.

Parenting Your Parents is also a book about hope. This book demonstrates that you're not alone—that hundreds of thousands of us face similar challenges every day, everywhere. We're all in this together, only we tend not to think of it that way. Most of us think that what we're facing is a singular, personal journey into the unknown. But the reality is that we all share a common responsibility of providing our parents with the love, care, support, affection, and attention they need and that we can deliver if we set our minds to it and plan now.

This is a book of hope, because it shares stories of others who are dealing with the same kinds of problems you're facing, or will face. It's a book of hope, because we help you plan for what you will have to consider and do at some point in time. And it's a book of hope, because it encourages you to think about the future and how to deal with it, rather than simply stand by and wait to be blindsided by the course of events. Finally, *Parenting Your Parents* is also a practical book, because it provides you with an extensive listing of organizations across the country that offer the kind of support and services you may need for your parents—or for yourself.

But it is not a book with all the answers. Seldom is anyone doing it all "the right way." What we bring you in this book are firsthand experiences, learned lessons to share, and many observations about the trauma, turmoil and challenges we're all facing or about to face.

As you read these words—at this very moment—a parent, somewhere, is in dire need of medical attention. And somewhere, a parent is dying. And somewhere else, a parent is about to fall and break a hip. And so it goes. So the story of our lives unfolds. None of us with parents is exempt from the process and consequences of the passage of time. It is a time to repay the profound debts we owe our parents who so much wanted us to forge and find our own good life.

Two days ago, my mother leaned on a dining room chair; it toppled and she fell. She was in pain all that night—especially her left arm—and the next morning the young woman who helps my parents took my mother to the emergency department of North York General Hospital. The X-ray showed a broken left wrist. Today, my mother is in bed with a cast to her elbow. She's being a real sport about it, but clearly she's in great discomfort and some pain. And she's confused by this new and unwanted experience. She doesn't yet know how to manage it. And she's looking for a lot of comforting support.

This morning I charged through the client work I had to do and then went to see her. She'd had a very bad night. So had my father. They both looked haggard. After all, my father, who has never fallen through all these years slipped in his bedroom just three weeks ago and fractured his left arm. He was in a cast from shoulder to fingers for 10 long, dreary days. His cast came off only five days before my mother's fall. They'd just begun to return to their routines, and now they are faced with her being in a cast for an estimated five weeks.

So I went to visit and help. I first helped my mother get out of bed, and it pained me to watch how uncertain she was when she finally stood and took a few tentative, wobbly steps. Determined, she walked the length of the hallway to the dining room, and then she wanted to get back into bed. We got all that done while my father finished dressing, and by that time he wanted to sit down for a short rest. And while he was calling me with questions about this and that, my mother was talking to me about her condition. But since both are now hard of hearing, they were competing for my attention without either knowing it. After dashing back and forth to listen—and respond—to both of them, I got them as settled and comfortable as possible.

Then I went grocery shopping for them. I looked for and selected things they really like, and especially those that are easily prepared. Knowing that my mother wouldn't be able to do much in the way of cooking or serving meals, I decided to make sure they were stocked with things I knew my father liked a lot and would easily prepare, and things I knew my mother liked to munch on. After showing my father what I had bought and storing everything where it belonged, I told my mother about my purchases so she'd know, and then I again helped her up and got her to sit at the kitchen table for a meal their helper was preparing.

Then I left for the day. This evening I called to see how they were doing. My mother said they were tired, but stable. Tomorrow, I will go to see them and help as best I can for a while. But now I will work on client projects in order to catch up and stay on top of what I need to do for our business. It's close to midnight. But I'm juggling. Balancing my work world responsibilities with what I feel are my responsibilities to my parents.

My partner in life and work, Gail, understands and is hugely supportive. But it's very evident that if we didn't have our own business, caring for my parents would be immensely difficult, if not impossible. As it is, we aren't as productive in our business as we could be because for the past few months I've been spending about 15 to 20 hours a week helping my parents. Gail's sensitivity stems from losing her mother to an obscure disease at an early age—in her mid-sixties—more than a decade ago, and from losing her father to cancer four years ago. Those painful events are still vivid in our minds and hearts, but even more so in hers.

Having our own business gives me the freedom and room to help my parents in a way that wouldn't be possible if I had a traditional corporate job. In fact, I remember seeing a news story that said research has shown that many people are losing opportunities for career advancement because they're passing on training and being overlooked for promotions since they need time off for parent care. That reminds me how long it took to get enlightened child care policies in the workplace, and it makes me wonder how long it will be before organizations become respectful and sensitive to the reality of the other end of life's spectrum and allow room in the working day for eldercare.

Meanwhile, Gail and I are living in a perpetual state of anticipation, concern, and, frankly, fear. Fear of the inevitable. Fear that we didn't do something we should have done. Concern that my parents have all they need to be comfortable. And the sad anticipation that at some point, some day, one of them will die, and we will need the strength and ability to help the surviving one, and ourselves, to face the future.

The lesson to be learned? There's nothing pretty about any of this. It's the drama of life and death. It's why we're here on the good planet Earth as human beings with emotions and values and passion.

It starts with the aging of our parents. It progresses through various stages of their needs, and the need for our support. It creates demands for which, for the most part, we're unprepared. Every step of the way, we come to realize how fragile we are and how frightening this journey really is.

And on this journey, nothing is clear or certain. Nothing is a given. There are no definite timelines or rules. Only, perhaps, that as the aging children of aging parents, we have a very difficult and critical and loving role to play. It's all about obligations and expectations — those of our parents and of ourselves.

It's all about finding coping mechanisms that allow us to do the best we can, to make our parents' lives as comfortable and meaningful as possible, while managing to have a life of our own.

It's all about learning how to help, but also about the limits of help without feeling guilt.

It's all about compassion and caring, and finding a way and means, while not losing ourselves in the process, to support those very parents who for so long did so much for us, and who now need us to do so much for them.

And that's precisely what we explore in this book. We give you a roadmap to build your confidence — to show you that you're far from being alone on what you may have thought was a lonely passage into the realm of caring for and helping your parents through their time of need.

Bart Mindszenthy

INTRODUCTION

The Rocky Road of Responsibility

KELLY , A FRIEND OF MANY YEARS, LEANS across the pub table with a beer in hand and says: "All our lives, we have this relationship with our parents where we expect them to be there, and we just don't talk about what would happen if things really change, if they're not there in the same way, and what we need to do, and how we plan for that."

I ponder Kelly's thought. He's right. We all face the same dilemma.

We talk some more about parents. How they're so much a part of our lives. How we both know them, and we don't. How we're both close, but not. How we think we'll be able to to manage the process of supporting them, but when push comes to shove, there are so many unknowns along the course of life that we more often than not don't know what to do or how to do it the best way.

We're not talking about parents dying. We're talking about parents at the end game of their lives, when their mental and physical capabilities are in rapid and steady decline. When from seemingly one day to the next, we—the children of our parents—find that we're cast into an uncharted and unwelcome role of caregivers to our parents.

A few beers later, we agree that our world is different. The old world was one where families were generally closer; where the care of fathers and mothers was easier just two generations ago because usually the mother didn't work outside the home and was a mainstay in helping parents while juggling responsibilities with children. But for better or for worse, that's not today's world. Women take a much more active part in the world of work outside the home, even while continuing to carry much of the responsibility of homemaking and child rearing. And often, they are the primary if not exclusive caregivers to their parents and sometimes even their in-laws. However, more and more, sons and sons-in-law are taking on these roles as well, and the world of work and new family structures are undergoing many confusing, contemporary changes.

We also talk about how aging parents have demands that are difficult to meet. As they age, our parents seem to simultaneously push and pull: push us away with outlandish views, and pull us closer with their needs and increasingly frequent voyages into their precious memories of the past in which we play a dominant role. For as they age, our parents seem to find comfort in the distant past and like to recall the many good and funny and emotional experiences we shared those many years ago.

As Kelly and I ponder these thoughts, I can't help but think about what hundreds of friends and acquaintances have told me over the past months since Michael and I started working on this book. All of them, when learning that we were working on a book called *Parenting Your Parents*, have been amazingly open in wanting to share their own experiences, worries, challenges, and trepidation. Frankly, I'm astounded by the candour of people who seem keen to talk about how they're trying to help their parents while managing their own day-to-day lives.

People's stories range from the sad to the humorous, and include weird and wonderful anecdotes about the real-life situations they're all facing. What they all have in common is the commitment to support their parents in any way they can, and the fact that doing so isn't easy or comfortable or clear.

The very next day after my evening out with Kelly, I get a call from Brian, a friend in Vancouver. During the course of our conversation, Brian talks about the difficulty of dealing with his parents as they age. Both are 86 years old, Brian reports, and it's so very difficult to listen to them and to help them. His father, who is blind, is very demanding. He wants meals at a certain time; he wants attention and help in a certain way. He wants many things, and expects to get them when he thinks it's best for him. Brian's mother has been coping as best she can, but not long ago, she simply collapsed from exhaustion. Brian had her admitted to a hospital and then made sure she stayed there for a week just to get a break and a rest from being the principal caregiver to her husband, while no one was principal caregiver to her. The week helped, but Brian is worried that his mother may collapse again given the strain of supporting her husband with no relief in sight.

Then I talk to good friend and business associate Judith in Toronto. Her father died two years ago, and last year, after a lot of researching she located a good seniors' home for her mother. Now her mother is happy with her setting. Judith visits regularly, helps her mother with her financial matters, and shares a special time once a week over a late afternoon cocktail and dinner. This is a time they both relish, savour and look forward to, and a time when Judith can carefully observe her mother to catch any changes that need to be considered.

Judith and her mother are fortunate because they can lead relatively normal lives and share the best with each other. Yet Judith is cautious and careful, making certain that her mother is both comfortable and secure on all counts, while fully cognizant that down the line her mother's condition will deteriorate. What Judith seems to be doing right is planning ahead and staying in close touch with her mother and the caregivers at the retirement home where her mother lives.

Shortly afterwards, my long-time friend Françoise, now living in the Eastern Townships southeast of Montreal, calls to check in. During our conversation, she tells me that her aging father is still as unpredictable as ever, and how frustrating it is to visit him on days when he either can't remember—or elects not to remember—what's happening or why. Her father has been drinking more than he should for some time now, and no matter how hard Françoise and her sister try, they can't get him away from the habit, which sometimes causes embarrassing and difficult family get-togethers.

This conversation makes me think of my partner's father who was highly unpredictable and loved his independence until his bout with cancer. I remember how Gail's family dealt with his death. How for many months we watched him slide ever lower, all the way fighting the concept of death, using every ounce of his energy to stay lucid and alive.

All this, while Gail and her brother arranged for every needed in-home service available to make their father as comfortable as possible while his pain grew day by day.

And there are so many others, all with a common concern, fear, confusion, and anxiety: how to support, help, and deal with aging parents. How to do what's right, while balancing a demanding life with their own families in a world that's moving too fast, and where all the rules are changing all the time.

Many of us feel enormous love and gratitude for what our parents have given to us and for the many sacrifices that they made throughout their lives for us. Some emigrated so that their children could live better lives. Some worked at more than one job to assure their children of a more comfortable life. Others took risks at work in order to improve their standard of living so that their children could study and find good jobs. Now it's our turn to care for them as they have cared for us: to care with love and devotion, even when the struggles and the challenges are sometimes overwhelming as we try to live our lives while we help our parents live their own lives to the fullest.

All the people I have talked to have poignant, intimate, emotional stories that are embedded in a not-too-distant past that is still vivid in their mind's eye. All of them wonder what they might have done differently to make the outcome better, more fulfilling, and less painful. And all of them regret that somehow, in some way, they couldn't have made it easier on everyone.

Listening hard, I realize that there is a consistent set of observations and frustrations that emerge:

- Parents have high expectations of receiving attention and all the things they think they want, and low tolerance for events and those things they want to ignore or avoid.
- Parents usually choose to remember being right and doing the right thing.
- Parents think we, their children, stay children, no matter what our age.

- Parents will try to protect us even while expecting us to help when necessary.
- Parents don't want to lose influence over us.
- Parents don't want to lose their sense of independence or dignity.
- Parents who are still together will defend each other with passion, even if they know that one of them has erred.
- Parents who have problems in their relationship with each other continue to have those problems even as they age; sometimes the issues become caricatures of their younger years.
- Parents, as they age and become more fragile, will rationalize their thinking and actions for fear of losing personal and family control.
- Parents see the world as they want, and there's nothing we can do to change that.
- Parents usually don't want to admit until it's too late that they need to rely on us, at which point we're usually frustrated and unsure how we can deliver the support they need.

So it's not an easy challenge that we, the children of our parents, face when we become by default the caregivers of our parents. Their wants and needs are demanding, and our ability to deliver is usually limited by time, resources, and priorities. Even when we want to give more, we are often in a conflict with the other demands on our lives — from our spouses, our children, and our work. There is an ongoing battle within us between meeting the demands or our daily lives and meeting our parents' needs.

But as Michael cautions throughout this book, this continuing internal battle can lead to problems if we don't measure carefully what we are realistically able to do, even when taking all the necessary steps to succeed. If we are not careful in how we pace and control what we are able to do, we can set ourselves up for terrible failure and risk undermining our own well-being and ability to successfully care for our parents. If we don't balance all the demands of our lives, we'll likely short-circuit ourselves along the way. We'll suffer mentally, and maybe even physically. And if that happens, we won't be much good to anyone—our spouse, our children, our parents, our employers, or ourselves. That's why we need to step back, assess, and take inventory about what we need to do to plan for and implement a sound, firm, logical strategy for helping our parents effectively and lovingly.

What we're into, in fact, is a delicate, difficult phase of our lives. There are no easy answers or magical solutions. The reality is that we'll all suffer, but at times we will also grow as we find new strength in our accomplishments. We need to try to maximize the small satisfactions and minimize the anguish and pain which often occurs as part of the aging process of our parents. At the end of the day, we should be able to say that we did what we could and were fortunate enough to have had the opportunity to care for our aging parents, through all the challenges and difficulties, and be better children and adults from the experience.

Another reality is that despite the challenges, we're expressing love and affection for our parents. We're showing them the respect and support they need and have every right to expect. We're simply balancing the scorecard of life. Because when we sit back dispassionately and take a lifelong inventory, chances are we'll find that in all the years since we were born, our parents did an awful lot for us. No doubt, we can all remember bad experiences. But the good experiences, and the good intent, almost always far outweighs the bad.

Caring for our parents can be tough and trying, yet if we really do love them for who they are and what they've tried to do for us, then it's a natural, healthy, and important commitment to make and take seriously. And no matter how hard things get—how trying—what must drive us is the wish and will to give our parents the comfort and dignity they deserve. So while our heads may stay pragmatic, our hearts will drive us to help them through the most difficult, demanding times. Because, bluntly put, that's the way life works. And that's of what each one of us with children hope will be the case when we're in need—even if we don't admit it.

CHAPTER ONE

Control:
Laying on the Guilt Trip

*FOR WHATEVER REASON, SOME PARENTS FIND it necessary to induce a sense
of guilt in their children, and even grandchildren, making relations difficult and
sometimes strained. This situation demands careful planning in order to defuse an
already delicate situation.*

The Challenge

Beth and Lloyd Thurmont are 83 and 86 years old respectively. They have
three children—Darrin, who is 58; Donna, 56; and Cameron, 54. Beth and
Lloyd live in a retirement home on the outskirts of Orangeville, Ontario.

Darrin, a chartered accountant, lives with his family in Brampton (a
45-minute drive away). He and his wife, Betty, have four children: 30-
year-old twin sisters Tracy and Tammy; Tom, who is 28 and lives in
London, Ontario with his wife, Angela, and their four children; and 26-
year-old Terry, who lives in Toronto with her lesbian partner.

Donna's marriage fell apart two years ago when her husband
announced he was leaving for another job in Vancouver and wanted to
start life over again. They have one child, Arthur, who at 38 goes from
job to job and city to city and who is still looking for a career path that

suits him. Donna now lives in a downtown Toronto bachelor apartment and works as a paralegal at a large law firm.

Cameron lives in Berlin, Germany, where he's been working as a freelance artist for the past five years. He enjoys his work and where he lives immensely. Single and unattached, Cameron loves roaming around Europe and has been back to Canada only twice to visit family and friends. He does call his parents about twice a month, and he sends them e-mail messages through his brother, Darrin.

Lloyd has been in ailing health for some years and is visited regularly by a nurse arranged through Ontario's Community Care Access Centre services, as well as by a physiotherapist who helps him exercise his severely arthritic legs and arms. Beth is in relatively good health, except for Type 2 diabetes, controlled by medication, and a weight problem she's had for decades.

Beth longs to have her children pay more attention to her and Lloyd and to see more of her grandchildren. No matter how much attention her family pays to her and Lloyd, for Beth it's not enough. She believes that in their old age, she and her husband are entitled to as much of their children's and grandchildren's time as they want and need.

In fact, in the past few years Beth has been exerting a steadily increasing level of control over her family by playing on their fears and instilling feelings of guilt. This has led to instances of both capitulation and confrontation among her children. Sometimes they've given in to the pressures placed on them, and sometimes they've had violent verbal battles. But most often, they've acquiesced in order to keep the peace and because their father always asks them to bear their mother's insecurities and to put up with her needs.

But now Beth's claims and attacks are more frequent and her needs more intense. She often calls with pleas for a quick appearance by one of her children because, she claims, Lloyd is desperate to see Darrin or Donna —usually a surprise to Lloyd, who is content to watch movies and read magazines most of the time. Or every so often she attacks Donna for failing in her marriage and causing embarrassment and grief for the whole family. Meanwhile, she alleges that Cameron rarely visits because he is selfish and has elected to escape his family responsibilities and that he lives a decadent life far away while everyone else is close to home and willing to help. And Darrin, she says, is guilty of putting his family before his parents because he only visits for an hour or so once or twice a week.

Beth is scathing in her views of her grandchildren who, she alleges, are only waiting to inherit the small fortune she and Lloyd have managed to save through years of back-breaking work. (The truth is, Beth and Lloyd are not very well off, and their three children actually contribute to offset the cost of living in the retirement home.) She often tells her children that they, like her grandchildren, would be smart to be nicer to her and Lloyd or they may lose their inheritance in favour of some worthy cause. And ever since Beth discovered that Terry was a lesbian, she's regularly harassed Darrin and Betty about it, telling them that if she were Terry's mother, this would never have happened. Terry, not surprisingly, has refused to see her grandmother for several years. Beth's other grandchildren tend to avoid any interaction with her, although they do confess to their parents that they would like to visit Lloyd alone, if that were possible.

No matter what responses her children give, Beth counters all of them with emotional outpourings and claims of feeling unwell or rejected. She works very hard at making all her children feel guilty in different ways.

For Beth's birthday in January, Darrin came to collect her and Lloyd and take them to his Brampton home, where Betty had prepared a lavish dinner. All four of Darrin and Betty's children attended, as did Donna. But by midway through dinner, everyone was miserable, as Beth spent considerable time telling stories about how durning the past year she and Lloyd had been disappointed and hurt by their children's insensitivity and their grandchildren's poor behaviour. The event turned into a painful experience for all of them, and at one point Donna got into a bitter exchange with her mother that left all of them hurt and embarrassed.

When she hasn't slept well for a couple of nights, or when she's feeling especially lonely and depressed, Beth calls her children and becomes agitated and confrontational in her tone and the content of her message, which is almost always the same: "What are you doing for me today?" Now, it's reaching the point where her children want to rebel and find ways to contain her outrageous claims, accusations, and anger.

Meanwhile, Lloyd continues to distance himself from the tension the family is feeling. For whatever reason, when he does talk to his children, it's always in a remote way that seems to imply his disinterest in his wife's needs and intensity. Lloyd, when he does see one of his children or talk to one of his grandchildren, usually discusses some movie or a television special he's seen, or an article he's read in *Reader's Digest*. And when he talks about Beth and her behaviour, it's usually in a very passive way, simply asking them to be understanding and to ignore her accusations.

> *The reality is that Darrin and Donna are having an increasingly difficult time coping with their mother's attitude and outbursts.*

But the reality is that Darrin and Donna are having an increasingly difficult time coping with their mother's attitude and outbursts. And since they can't detect any certain signs of mental illness or any other problem, they are confused and frustrated. They relay their impressions to Cameron, who says he just isn't close enough to be able to pass judgment.

Darrin recently spoke to his parents' family physician who said that there doesn't seem to be anything wrong with Beth. In fact, she seems relatively well, generally upbeat, and positive about her life, but she has expressed concerns that her children and grandchildren are ignoring Lloyd, and this she finds hurtful and wrong. She told the doctor that Lloyd suffers as a result and that, in turn, she's stressed. The doctor told Darrin that Beth did volunteer that she misses more interaction with her children and grandchildren, and that she does believe that all of them would just as soon see her and Lloyd dead and gone so they wouldn't have to care about them.

Darrin, in sharing this information with Donna and Cameron, also tells them that he feels their parents' doctor sympathizes with their mother's sense of being wronged. He tells them he's concerned that the doctor is, for whatever reason, biased in her favour, and that as a result he's not being as helpful as he should be in either assessing her or prescribing some kind of medication to manage her moods.

The Health Care Professional's Point of View

This is the kind of difficult family dynamic that can either lead to further family disruption with a permanent legacy of hurt and guilt, or one that can bring a family together and demonstrate how robust they are in dealing with difficult situations. Most families at times have to face trying situations that may test the very fabric of family ties. Whether it is illness, death, terrible financial situations or complex family dynamics, there are ways of resolving issues so that irremediable damage does not occur.

We can work on the assumption that there is nothing wrong with Beth medically that may account for her increasing need for family attention and that what is occurring is merely a manifestation of her underlying personality. Even though the family physician may not be impressed that there is anything wrong with her, it may be worthwhile for a family spokesperson to speak to the doctor and question whether, indeed, something underlying might be going on. Sometimes conditions such as depression or early dementia result in peculiar exaggerations of personality. This possibility can be addressed by the family physician by probing for symptoms and conducting mental-status testing. If the physician is sure that what is going on is not related to an underlying clinical condition, then Beth has to be dealt with as a full participant in whatever process might be developed to help resolve this increasingly tense and potentially destructive situation.

To assist the family and Beth and Lloyd, a two-part process can be implemented. First, the children, especially the two in Ontario, need to get some help in sorting through this very challenging situation. If this is not done in some cohesive fashion, the result could be terrible alienation of the various members of the family that is likely to have long-lasting effects on the family structure. It is important that the grandchildren who live in the vicinity also take part in the process, as the patterns of family interaction, the value put on relationships, and the ability to deal with difficulty are often measures of a family's strength for the present and the future.

One approach is to find a social worker (or some other family counsellor) who is experienced in dealing with issues of family dynamics. It is important to define who the key players will be in any family meetings that take place initially to try and provide a framework for the issues, problems, and options. But, even for those who do not actually attend family sessions, there must be consistent communication so that everyone is "on board" with the approach. This is an opportunity for all the children to address the issues and, if at all possible, to be consistent with the approach to their parents (and grandparents).

Assuming that such family counselling takes place, the second part of the process is to have a clear discussion with Beth and Lloyd about what is going on. There may be a number of ways of doing this, including having the key members of the family meet with Beth and Lloyd alone (not too many in the first meeting, but clearly representing the consensus of the family) and explaining the enormous difficulties that everyone is facing. It makes sense to begin a meeting of this sort with a clear statement of the love, devotion, and commitment that the family has for their parents, but that the ability to carry out their own complex lives and at the same time respond to every whim and need of Beth may not be possible.

Of course at this point, it is possible that Beth may become very upset or angry at "being ganged up on," and she may not want any further part of the discussions. If this happens, it would be time for one person, perhaps Darrin, to speak to his mother again and continue with the same message: "We love you and dad, and want only the best for you, but...," laying out the difficulties that everyone is facing. It must be made clear to Beth that when she insults her children and grandchildren it is having the opposite effect to the one she hopes to achieve.

It might be suggested to Beth and Lloyd (or to Beth alone if that seems preferable) that she join a few of the family with the counsellor. If she agrees, that is a major step forward. If she rejects that offer, it still may be possible to work with her and Lloyd to find an acceptable and agreeable common ground.

Some of the arrangements that sometimes work in such situations include developing a rotation system of who will visit or communicate with whom on a regular basis. There may be some need to increase the interaction of the family with Lloyd and Beth, but rather than being on an "on-call" basis, the family could put together an outline of what can and cannot be done reasonably within clearly defined limits.

Someone should make it clear that there are no financial expectations from Beth and Lloyd, and if, indeed, the children are paying for some of the expenses, this can be pointed out. Most important, it must be related to Beth, either by a family member (or two) or by a counsellor, that the family fabric is being disrupted because of the recriminations and accusations that may ultimately cause the family network and ties to unravel. That would be the worst outcome possible because eventually

Beth and Lloyd may have needs that will require a great deal of devotion and time, and an enormous sense guilt may follow the family members for years to come.

Family dynamics are among the most difficult issues to challenge. But the children and grandchildren have to come to terms with the long-haul implications of decisions they make. Families are not replaced by other entities, and it is worth the investment to try and salvage whatever relationships exist for the immediate situation and for the future. There are ways of learning how not to react to hurtful words when it is clear that the result will be counterproductive. There are ways for Beth's family to consistently remind her that her family loves her, but that she must find better ways to help them carry out their love than trying to bully them into it.

> *Family dynamics are among the most difficult issues to challenge. But the children and grandchildren have to come to terms with the long-haul implications of decisions they make.*

CHAPTER TWO

Surgery:
Weighing the Odds

SURGERY AT ANY AGE CAN BE TRAUMATIC, but for elderly parents, there are special issues and considerations. Weighing priorities and planning recovery is a complex and demanding process requiring careful consideration.

The Challenge

Lee Ann Bowater is 76 and a widow. Her husband, Martin, died four years ago after suffering several heart attacks. She lives alone in a one-bedroom apartment in Halifax, and while she still mourns Martin's death, she has moved on with her life. Lee Ann has several friends, and they try to get together at least once a week for tea and talk.

Lee Ann's daughter, Sylvia, is an elementary school teacher. She's 52 years old and lives in Dartmouth with her husband, Gerry, who works long hours managing a car rental outlet in downtown Halifax. Sylvia and Gerry have two children: Jay, age 28, and Linda, age 19. Jay moved to Moncton three years ago to work in a call centre, and Linda lives at home as she continues her education at a local college.

Lee Ann's son, David, is 47 years old and lives in Calgary, where he works as an analyst for an oil company. He divorced two years ago and lives in an apartment with his common-law partner, Mary, whom Lee Ann has never met.

Both children are in close contact with Lee Ann, especially Sylvia, who lives only 12 kilometres away and visits her mother every other day. As well, every two weeks, Gerry picks up Lee Ann to take her to their home for dinner. David calls from Calgary at least once a week to talk to his mother for a few minutes, and he tries to visit at least once a year.

Lee Ann relishes visits from her daughter, and she tries hard to be a loving, non-intrusive grandmother to Jay and Linda, although she considers both to be somewhat spoiled. However, she works very hard at keeping those feelings to herself, and she spends most of the time during Sylvia's visits asking about her teaching and Gerry's work.

Lee Ann is relatively sound in body and mind. She is short and a bit overweight, but not so much that it's a problem. In fact, since Martin's death, she has shown a surprisingly strong sense of independence, and has learned to manage her finances so that Gerry only needs to spend an hour a month reviewing her bank statements.

Five years ago Lee Ann had surgery for cataracts in both eyes. This was a low-risk, high-benefit proposition that allowed her to again see well and resume a relatively normal lifestyle. In fact, she found she once again could play canasta with her friends.

Now, however, Lee Ann has developed a malignant tumour in her colon that is still relatively small, but has the potential to grow and spread. Her doctor believes surgery will be required at some point. As well, she is in constant pain because of severe osteoarthritis in her left hip, and a hip replacement operation is the only certain way to help her with that condition.

Lee Ann's doctor is cautious about the prognosis, noting that while the operations are fairly routine, Lee Ann will need substantial support for a prolonged period of time afterward. The hip operation is not critical, but would allow Lee Ann to walk and function more easily and would probably eliminate the pain with which she's living. The colon surgery, on the other hand, is more urgent because of the risk of the tumour spreading.

Lee Ann understands that she needs the colon surgery, and she also wants the hip replacement, but she is fearful of the two operations and the period of convalescence. It's clear that if either operation is to proceed, Lee Ann will require close, ongoing help and support during her recovery.

Sylvia knows that her mother would like to live with her and Gerry during her recovery. Gerry is against this idea because they live in a small house with two bedrooms, and they both work full time. While he hasn't said "no" to the prospect of Lee Ann living with them, it is not an option he would happily embrace.

David has said that he wants to be supportive, but that distance prevents him from doing much in terms of hands-on help.

Given Lee Ann's limited income, as well as the limited incomes of both Sylvia and David, there is no clear resolution to the question of how the family will support her.

> *The challenge for the family is how to help Lee Ann face two surgical procedures, both of which are necessary to give her the chance of survival and an improved quality of life. How can they help without disrupting their own equilibrium in an unacceptable way?*

The challenge for the family is how to help Lee Ann face two surgical procedures, both of which are necessary to give her the chance of survival and an improved quality of life. How can they help without disrupting their own equilibrium in an unacceptable way?

The family faces several important issues. Should the colon surgery be performed first? If so, that would require at least two or three weeks of in-home care. But where should Lee Ann stay for that period of time? If she were to remain in her apartment, she would require professional home care services, as well as someone to live with her during her convalescence. Or, could Lee Ann stay with Sylvia and her family, or with David and his partner? Could David take off a few weeks and stay with his mother?

If the colon surgery is performed first and Lee Ann has a good recovery, then should the orthopaedic surgery be undertaken to replace her left hip? And if so, when? Rehabilitation work would be necessary after the hip surgery, and that would mean Lee Ann would have to be taken for rehab sessions at least twice a week for several weeks.

Sylvia and Gerry have talked about what they could and should do. Their daughter, Linda, has made it clear that she won't have time to help because of her school and social commitments. Their son, Jay, is relatively independent but works long hours. Sylvia herself is concerned about any surgery during the school year, because she won't be able to take the kind of time off that would probably be required. And Gerry, given the nature of his job, can't be counted on for any extended level of support.

Sylvia has also discussed the situation with her brother during the course of several telephone conversations. She's even suggested that David take his holidays and spend two weeks with their mother after the colon operation to help her. David listened to the case Sylvia presented, but responded by saying that Mary was really counting on having their holidays together for a long-planned drive to tour the Grand Canyon and to spend time in Las Vegas. This has irritated Sylvia, but the siblings have both stayed very polite with each other.

Lee Ann's doctor, in a recent telephone call with Sylvia, advised that while he wants to do some further tests, he believes the colon surgery will be imperative based on the steady growth of the tumour. He tells Sylvia that "sooner than later" is the way they should think about it.

The Health Care Professional's Point of View

Lee Ann and her family have a few things to figure out and a real examination of relationships and priorities is in order for this situation to work well. It is worth dividing the issues into those that are mainly clinical and those that are related to the way the family feels it should and can support Lee Ann, who wants to remain independent, but who is facing some difficult challenges in the next little while.

When considering the clinical issues, the priority is likely going to be the removal of the colon tumour. From the information provided, it appears that the tumour is still at a stage where if removed surgically, a good outcome is likely and Lee Ann should be able to function independently. It is worth asking the surgeon if the surgery can be done in such a way that bowel function will be maintained and that a colostomy (exit of bowel through the skin) will not be required. The answer will have a big impact on the type of care required immediately after the surgery and for the longer term following.

Also, the assumption is that the tumour will be contained and will not spread (metastasize) to other organs, so that the outlook over a longer period of time would be good. However, until the surgery is done it is hard to know whether further treatments such as radiation therapy might be required.

The family must understand that there is some urgency to the decision about the colon surgery and that they must find ways to support their mother through this emotionally and physically trying situation. Although Lee Ann may be holding herself together in face of what is probably a very frightening prospect, that of cancer surgery, it appears that she does not want to be a burden on her family. This is the time for her children to find the means to rally around and support their mother, one way or another, within the resources, human and otherwise, that they have available.

They can look at the challenges in a few stages. The first is the immediate preparation for surgery with its emotional and physical impact. This is the time for everyone to find time, in a co-operative fashion, to be there to bolster their mother (and grandmother).

Assuming that all goes well, the stages following surgery will be divided into the immediate post-operative phase and then a period of Lee Ann's reactivation and return to a "normal" functioning lifestyle. It is important for the family to explore what assistance is available for their mother's post-surgical care to help all of them cope in terms of time limitations. Although such assistance often does not completely replace the need for family, it can provide proper care for the patient while families carry on with their other responsibilities. Reactivation programs in long-term care facilities may be available in some jurisdictions, although this is not always possible. Home care options, providing nursing care and some homemaking, may be available as part of the health care program. This may have to be supplemented through paid help in addition to whatever the family can weave together in order for their mother to get over the immediate post-operative and return-to-home period.

It would be worth exploring whether there are friends and neighbours available to give a little help. In fact, such help may very well be readily forthcoming and may pleasantly surprise the family and Lee Ann. Although the family may not want to impose on others, often neighbours and friends feel that helping out is one of the ways to demonstrate affection and caring, so asking for help should not be dismissed or declined out of hand.

It's a real challenge to families when they have to interrupt their busy lives to deal with a family crisis. But everyone in the family has to step back and ask, "Do I want my mother (grandmother, mother-in-law, etc.) to survive this ordeal?" After all, family should take a priority in times of difficulty, and major cancer surgery is just that kind of challenge.

Moving into Sylvia's home is probably not ideal given the cramped space, but if another arrangement cannot be made for the immediate period after surgery this option should be reconsidered. Families can usually find ways to come together during times of crisis and Lee Ann's surgery should be considered to be precisely that: a crisis in the making. Most employers are understanding when there is a family illness, and it may be necessary for family members to get some extra time off to help look after Lee Ann at Sylvia and Gerry's home until she feels secure enough to return to her own home with some home care in addition to what her family can provide.

As for David, this is a time to test his relationships. It would seem reasonable to expect of one's "significant other" to compromise on vacation plans if a family member's health is at stake. David's moving in with his mother for a week might make all the difference, with a little supplement from home care professionals and homemakers and input from other family members, including the grandchildren, in helping Lee Ann get over this difficult time. The way everyone comes together in this time of need will be a reflection of the fabric of this family. Anyone can be constructive and positive when there are no demands. It is when there are difficult times that families have their true strength tested, and for Lee Ann's family, this is one such time.

If Lee Ann gets through the colon surgery without much problem, the issue of her hip should be a lesser challenge. First, if the colon surgery goes well, this should help Lee Ann and her family understand the steps necessary to negotiate the health care and home care systems. Second, following major orthopaedic surgery, there are often programs in place to assist in the rehabilitation process.

It would be wise for Lee Ann to wait at least three months following the colon surgery before having the hip operation. This should give her ample time to regain her emotional and physical strength and her independence. If more time for recovery is required, then the hip surgery should be done later as the urgency for it is not great.

Lee Ann's family should inquire whether or not in-patient rehabilitation exists. If it does, arrangements should be made after discussions with the orthopaedic surgeon and if appropriate, the social service department of the hospital to make certain that the post-operative plan includes admission at an in-patient rehabilitation unit. If such an arrangement is possible (and it usually is), then Lee Ann's concerns about being a "burden" to her family and disrupting their lives change considerably. Following anywhere from four to six weeks on a rehabilitation unit, Lee Ann will in all likelihood be able to return home with minimal assistance.

Most rehabilitation programs provide some evaluation of the home setting and recommend or arrange for modifications to accommodate the patient's ability to function. If the hip replacement will make Lee Ann more independent than she was prior to surgery, it is likely that little, if anything, will have to be done to the home to meet her needs. However, some safety measures might be recommended, especially in the bathroom to make sure she can bathe safely and not risk falling.

If Lee Ann and her children are concerned about Lee Ann being alone in her home, they can look into an emergency response system, such as Lifeline (see the Resource Directory at the back of the book), which allows individuals to call for help should they fall or injure themselves, and which often provides an element of security to themselves and their families.

> *Illness poses a great challenge both to those affected by the illness and to their families. This is a special time for families to enrich their relationships and to demonstrate what they are willing and able to do for their loved one.*

Illness poses a great challenge both to those affected by the illness and to their families. This is a special time for families to enrich their relationships and to demonstrate what they are willing and able to do for their loved one. It has to be a co-operative affair so that there are no resentments that can linger and cause hard feelings later. What better way to demonstrate affection to a parent in special need, even the most independent parent, than to help as an act of love and devotion? That is what families are all about.

CHAPTER THREE

Independence:
Helping Parents Live Their Lives

SOMETIMES IN THEIR ZEAL TO HELP AND protect their parents, children add to their discomfort by making decisions that may be well intentioned, but actually serve to disrupt tried and true lifestyles. The result is increased family tension and parental angst.

The Challenge

Ivan and Sophie Bogdonovich immigrated to Canada in 1948. Their eventual arrival here is a story in itself. During the depths of World War II, Ivan, who had been unwillingly conscripted into the Soviet army, was injured and judged unfit for further service. He was, however, assigned to work in a factory several hundred kilometres from his village. After nearly a year at the factory, he managed to escape two months before the end of the war, work his way back to his village, and reunite for one night with his family and wife.

Under the deep cover of the next night, he and his young wife, Sophie, left their native village in the Ukraine with only the clothes on their backs and a satchel full of food. They managed to reach the Austrian boarder just as the war ended, and they were two of the first few to be accepted into an Austrian refugee camp where they were interned for three years. They applied to both the United States and Canada for refugee status, and eventually were linked through the Red Cross with a sponsor in Red Deer, Alberta. The sponsor was a distant relative who agreed to help them settle in Canada.

Ivan is now in his late seventies and Sophie is in her mid-seventies. (No one is certain of their ages, and there is no birth record that has ever been found.) They're in fairly good health, but starting to show signs of forgetfulness.

They have two sons: Boris, 49, who was born in the Austrian refugee camp just months before the family came to Canada, and Bob, 41, who was born in Red Deer. Both brothers left home some 20 years ago and they now both live in Montreal. Because the brothers are close to each other and comfortable with their lives in Montreal, they decided that to best help their parents, they should move them to a retirement home close to them.

At the time of this decision, neither parent really wanted to leave Red Deer, where they had a number of friends and an active social life. They were well known in the community because, from the mid-1950s to just two years ago, they operated a popular diner known for its spicy cabbage rolls, various potato soups, and other ethnic dishes. However, Boris and Bob were persistent. During their annual visits and weekly telephone calls, the brothers finally convinced their parents that to best care for them and in order to be close, they should move to Montreal.

Nine months later, Ivan and Sophie sold their home, shipped their belongings ahead, and a week later took the train to Montreal. They had been to Montreal a handful of times during the past 15 years to visit their sons, but they knew only a little about the city, which they considered somewhat intimidating in comparison to comfortably sized Red Deer. But as they got older, they also longed to be closer to their sons, and they knew of no other way than moving to make that possible.

Boris and Bob, who really are close to each other and very fond of their parents and proud of what they have done with their lives, were determined to make the move a good one. After considerable searching, they found a small but attractive one-bedroom apartment for their parents, which they agreed to subsidize.

To surprise their parents, Boris and Bob arranged to have their parents' furniture, clothing, kitchenware, and all other belongings, shipped and delivered to the apartment. They spent a full day putting the place in some kind of order that they thought would please their parents.

When Ivan and Sophie arrived, Boris and his wife, Janet, and Bob and his wife, Adele, and their two children, Jennifer, 12, and April, 10, met them at the station. Initially, there was much joy, and Sophie cried when she met her family and saw the new apartment, which was about equidistant from both sons' homes. She cried even more when she saw most of what was in her old home crammed into the small apartment. And so began a new life in a new place for Ivan and Sophie.

Now, months later, the euphoria of being reunited and living in the same city has waned. The first negative experience was when Ivan discovered that he was very intimidated driving in Montreal. The shear volume of traffic scared him, and he found himself easily confused by the bilingual signs everywhere. Yet driving was important to him; having a car and being able to drive was, for Ivan, an important symbol of his independence. Now he was hardly driving at all.

Both Ivan and Sophie have found that getting around the city without the help of their sons is difficult, if not impossible. To them, public transportation is intimidating. The subways are frightening, and they feel unsure of themselves on the escalators, in the subway cars, or even in knowing how to get to where they thought they wanted to go. In short, Ivan and Sophie feel lost and confused by Montreal's size and its very different culture. They miss their friends and the city that for so long was home and that they knew so well.

But worst for them is that they have a strong sense that Boris's and Bob's wives are resentful of the time their husbands spend with their parents. Neither Janet nor Adele call or come to visit very often, and when they do, or when Ivan and Sophie go to their homes for a visit or a meal, there is always a feeling of tension and discomfort. But just as hard to bear for Ivan and Sophie is that their two granddaughters are completely alien who show no interest in or respect for them.

When they spend any time at all with Jennifer and April, it's strained and unsatisfying.

After nearly nine months in Montreal, Ivan and Sophie are miserable, lonely, dejected, and depressed. They see their sons less frequently and are certain it's because the wives are exerting pressure on Boris and Bob—which, in fact, is the case.

Meanwhile, Janet and Adele continue to lobby their husbands for more of their time, and more time with their own parents. It's now become a subtle battle of wills—to see whose parents will get what level of attention.

Boris and Bob are confused; they thought they'd done the right thing, for all the right reasons. They're further agitated by the behaviour of their wives, which they'd never anticipated and can't fully understand.

Then, when their parents tell them they would rather return to Red Deer, the brothers are frustrated and angered. In their minds, they've been very responsible and logical, and they can't understand why their parents aren't contented and, in fact, grateful. Nor can they understand why their parents don't go out on their own more and meet people in the Ukrainian community. Both Boris and Bob have taken them to the Ukrainian Orthodox church in Montreal and to a Ukrainian social club, where they thought their parents would find some new friends.

> *Even though their health is slowly deteriorating, Ivan and Sophie are still capable of independent living, and they tell their sons that while they love them dearly, this arrangement isn't working out at all.*

But their parents are adamant about their unhappiness and desire to move back to Red Deer. Even though their health is slowly deteriorating, Ivan and Sophie are still capable of independent living, and they tell their sons that while they love them dearly, this arrangement isn't working out at all.

The Health Care Professional's Point of View

Nothing is as disappointing as disappointment. We often have imaginary views of what people are like and how we can create situations that will ensure their happiness or at least contentment. Anticipated emotions and fantasies are often very different from the actualities of everyday life. That is why everyone is disappointed in the outcome of Boris and Bob's plans for their parents and the reality that Ivan and Sophie are experiencing in their day-to-day life in Montreal.

Moving is hard for everyone and a new situation is often fraught with unknown situations and unanticipated responses. Whether a move is for work, study, or personal obligations, most people adapt out of necessity. And sometimes a move means immediate success — perhaps a better job, a nicer house, new challenges, and often new friends. But when a move happens later in life, it can be much more difficult. Most people's dearest friends are from the earlier years of life, and long-time bonding is not easily duplicated in later years. The shared memories and reference points for collective reminiscence, such an important part of social activity, is lost as the fabric of friends is disrupted by death or by a move away.

So what happened here with this clearly caring family, that might have been averted, and is there any way of salvaging the situation?

First of all, a decision to move an older relative must be made with careful thought. A family can rarely be a sufficient substitute for a social network. Families may care for loved ones more in the deepest sense, but they cannot replace the normal social activities with a familiar circle of friends in a long accustomed environment.

> *Families may care for loved ones more in the deepest sense, but they cannot replace the normal social activities with a familiar circle of friends in a long accustomed environment.*

Before considering the move, Boris and Bob should have discussed with their parents what it was that they thought they would need in order to be reasonably satisfied, if not happy, in Montreal. If all the answers were focused on the closeness of the family, everyone might have stepped back and asked, "Is that going to be enough?" Also, some frank discussion with spouses and children should have taken place in order to avoid feelings of hurt or abandonment. It is not always easy for a spouse or children to feel that their time is not "lost" when there is often so little time available for "normal" family relationships.

It might have been worthwhile to try out the arrangement, perhaps giving it a chance with a three- or four-month visit, using a rented apartment or house and not moving everything out right away. This would have given Ivan and Sophie an opportunity to figure out what there is in the new community that might be attractive enough to make the move worthwhile, separate from the anticipated need to be with family as their faculties decline and health becomes compromised.

If, after a prolonged visit, Sophie and Ivan felt that they would likely be isolated, perhaps a permanent move would not have been contemplated. Some families choose to have a number of prolonged visits to provide an opportunity to explore and make some acquaintances that might form the nucleus of new friendships should a permanent move be undertaken. The sons could not possibly fill the void left by the loss of the network that Ivan and Sophie had in Red Deer. Children are rarely friends with their parents, and the child-parent role is hard to change even in mature years.

For their part, Ivan and Sophie should have had a heart-to-heart talk with each other to understand why they decided to make the move. They needed to understand that while they would be losing some of their present enjoyment in Red Deer, they would at least be with family and feel secure should something go wrong. There is nothing wrong with that choice, but when they made it, they needed to decide to dedicate themselves to finding ways to make it work, rather than comparing their situation to what was before. Such a move could never result in their having the same social milieu that existed with their friends in Red Deer. But if they felt that the modest amount of loneliness and lack of social network was worth the investment in the future, then they might have come to terms with the trade-off. Clearly they had the strength during their younger years to make such a choice, but in later years, it was less easy to do.

Finally, Boris and Bob need not feel that they failed. They also cannot blame their families for letting their parents down. It would be an extraordinary family that could accept a major shift of attention from their lives to that of parents now living in the community whose needs are great, without some feeling of resentment. This would be true even when coupled with great filial dedication to care for one's parents and those of one's spouse.

Because things are not working out the family needs to explore the alternatives, the last one being that Ivan and Sophie be allowed to move back to Red Deer, either temporarily or permanently. A frank discussion with everyone in the family, without any blame or suggestion that someone is at "fault," might help clear the air. An external counsellor might help the discussion, but one is not necessary for this situation to be fully explored among everyone involved.

Sometimes people imagine the past as better than the present. Maybe, indeed, life would be better if Ivan and Sophie moved back to Red Deer. But, perhaps not. They may not be able to re-align themselves with their previous network. They could try moving back for a few months, renting a suitable place that would not require them to move all their belongings again. Or, they could decide as a family that the future was so risky for Ivan and Sophie that everyone is going to have to sacrifice a bit for things to work out.

Ivan and Sophie are going to have to sacrifice their illusion that life in Montreal is going to be as good as their life in Red Deer. They need to figure out what can they do to make it as good as possible. They clearly had the strength to make difficult moves in the past, and now they have to draw on their strength to do it again. They need to decide to "force" themselves to join activities or centres that might provide them with a new network of acquaintances and activities, even if they aren't ideal. The attitude in which they undertake that task will go a long way in terms of likely success. I have seen many of my patients resist any mention of joining a club or taking on a volunteer position only to thank me later because of the success of the outcome.

The wives and grandchildren have to come to some agreement about how they will deal with Ivan and Sophie living nearby. This should include the kind of time commitment that would be reasonable and acceptable, knowing that in all likelihood things will improve with time if everyone is very caring and supportive in the beginning. It is not too late to salvage the situation.

Boris and Bob should admit to their parents that they realize they made some mistakes moving them to Montreal, but tell them that there is a time to try and turn things around. And they should remind their parents that the reason for the decision to move in the first place was the concern that Ivan or Sophie, or both of them, might need help because of failing health. Bob and Boris would not be able to provide that help in Red Deer, and Ivan and Sophie could end up quite isolated in that community. Ivan and Sophie should agree to give the move another try, for about four months. During this time they could join some social groups and really try and see what might happen if they attempted to meet people and develop a new network of friends.

The agreement might be that if after four months of everyone trying their best to explore the relationship, build on its strengths, and understand the long-term benefits for the future, things are not better, Ivan and Sophie will move back to Red Deer. If so, Boris and Bob will not have failed, nor will have their families.

In due course the situation may resolve itself by Ivan and Sophie needing medical care in Red Deer and receiving it there, or progressively deteriorating so that they cannot look after themselves, but finding somewhere to stay in that community. Or, perhaps after one of the parents dies, the one who survives will accept that there are no real choices but to join their children again in Montreal.

No matter what decision is made, the important thing to remember is that this is not a failure, but merely a human attempt to be a loving family. Plans don't always turn out the way we would like them to, and that is just the way things are, even when those plans are made with the best of intentions.

CHAPTER FOUR

Breaking the Mold:
The Rebellious Grandmother

SOMETIMES WE MAKE ASSUMPTIONS ABOUT OUR parents that are wrong, and that can lead to negative consequences, as in this case of an elderly woman whose daughter mistakenly decides what her mother would like to do.

The Challenge

Fatima Campenello is a 74-year-old widow who never mastered English, despite living in Canada for 50 years. She and her husband, Julio, moved to Canada from their native Italy in 1952, the day after her 25th birthday. On arrival, they landed in Toronto's large Italian community, where for the first few years they lived in a one-bedroom apartment and started life anew.

Julio's cousin, who had come to Toronto several years earlier, already had a relatively good job in a bakery, and he helped Julio and Fatima settle in. While Julio soon landed a job working as a shipping dock hand at the city's food and produce terminal, Fatima found nothing after considerable searching . Eventually, though, she started cleaning homes in the area. She also spent considerable time babysitting for neighbours and even for some of the clients for whom she cleaned. And so cleaning and looking after young children became her full-time work for many years.

In 1964, when Fatima was 37 and Julio 42, Fatima became pregnant and gave birth to their only child, Angela. While both were delighted at the arrival of the child, it was a surprise coming fairly late in their lives. Fatima lavished time and attention on her daughter while still working five days a week cleaning homes and babysitting. If she had to babysit in the evenings, she'd often take Angela along so she could spend time with her daughter, and her daughter could play with new friends.

Eventually, the Campenellos moved into a two-bedroom unit of a fourplex, still in Toronto's Italian community. Twice they made the pilgrimage back their old hometown in southern Italy, and over the years a few relatives came to visit them.

Angela thrived in school and revelled in her cultural heritage. She learned to speak fluent Italian and to read and write in the language. Her English was also flawless. She graduated with honours from high school and went on to earn a university degree in psychology with top grades. Once she finished her schooling, she found a job in a teen counselling centre. In her late twenties, Angela married Frank Combriani, a hardworking chartered accountant whose parents had also emigrated from Italy in the early 1950s. For the first few years of their marriage, Angela and Frank lived in a downtown apartment, and then bought a small house in suburban Scarborough. When Julio retired at age 66, Fatima continued to babysit a few half days a week. The extra income was welcome and she enjoyed the work. Over the years she had gained a strong reputation for her skill with children. In fact, she was babysitting the children of some of those she babysat years earlier. In their increasing free time, Julio and Fatima socialized, still staying for the most part in their Italian community.

Four years ago, Julio, who'd complained with increasing frequency about headaches but who refused for the longest time to see a doctor, was diagnosed with a brain tumour. Surgery was determined to be too risky, and his age further compounded the situation. Julio died two years ago.

For a period of time after his death, Fatima continued to live on her own in their small home, but found it increasingly difficult to manage. She explored the option of finding another woman to share the house with, but that seemed complicated. She considered moving into a retirement home, but because she was in relatively good health, the notion of being around so many "old people" left her thinking that wasn't such a good idea.

That's when Angela and Frank suggested to her that she move in with them. By this time they had a five-year-old son, Frank Jr., who was about to start kindergarten, but they had a large enough house that included a small, self-contained apartment in the basement. After much discussion and a lot of thinking, Fatima decided that perhaps it would be a good move. She loved her daughter, and she was very fond of Frank. A month later, she made the move.

Generally, the transition was good. Fatima liked her little room and her privacy, and she also liked spending some time with her grandson. She especially liked her time with her daughter and son-in-law, because they could speak comfortably in Italian. She would also watch a considerable amount of Italian television programming, and every few weeks Frank or Angela would take her to visit some of her friends in her old neighbourhood.

Then Angela became pregnant again and delivered a very healthy, beautiful daughter, Gabriella—which soon became "Gabby." Angela took six months off work to be home with Gabby, and life seemed to be good for all. When it was time for Angela to go back to work, she asked her mother to babysit Gabby, since she was living with them anyway, and it was clear she liked spending time with her. Fatima seemed reluctant, but she did agree, and so Angela didn't give it any further thought as she resumed her work life.

As the months passed, both Frank and Angela noticed that Fatima seemed more withdrawn and, as they saw it, depressed. However, whenever they asked Fatima if there was a problem or if she felt well, the response was always the same: a firm denial that anything was wrong, end of conversation. Yet neither Frank nor Angela could accept Fatima's protests as they could see that her day-to-day behaviour was becoming evermore inwardly focused.

Finally, Angela called a nearby geriatric clinic and arranged for an assessment, and then broke the news to her mother. She told her mother that she was simply worried about her, and disguised her true concern by explaining that given her age, Fatima needed to be seen by those specializing in the health of the elderly.

Mother and daughter went to the clinic for the appointment. The geriatrician first met with both Fatima and Angela, who explained to the doctor that her mother seemed increasingly depressed. She shared that her mother was withdrawn and preferred to spend more and more time in her room, whereas just months ago she seemed to really enjoy family interaction and playing with her grandchildren. Fatima did not contradict her daughter's depiction of the situation.

Then the physician started his examination of Fatima alone, during which time he asked her what was going on from her perspective. He noted that he could not find anything physically wrong with her but was concerned about her mood. He told her she seemed down and "blue." Although her English was not perfect, Fatima was able to express herself adequately to explain that she didn't want to babysit her new granddaughter. Fatima explained that she'd been looking after people's children and homes for most of her life, and that she was tired of looking after others—whether they were children or adults.

She said she loved her grandchildren, but she wanted to enjoy them and not feel like she had to work at it five days a week.

She said she loved her grandchildren, but she wanted to enjoy them and not feel like she had to work at it five days a week. The geriatrician told her that she had to be honest with her daughter about her feelings but Fatima initially balked, saying she did not want to hurt her daughter whom she loved very much. The doctor said he would help her explain and that everything would be all right.

When the geriatrician told Angela what Fatima had said, Angela was shocked. She and Frank had assumed that because her mother spent so much time babysitting over the years that she'd be very comfortable continuing in that role with her own grandchildren. Plus, they trusted Fatima with Gabby and Frank Jr. And, truth be known, the arrangement helped them reduce expenses. But mostly, Angela said, it was their belief that her mother would thrive in looking after her grandchildren; this, after all, is what both remembered seeing so much of in their old Italian neighbourhood in their own youth. Angela expressed regret that she had put her mother in this unfair situation and said she wanted to help resolve the situation in any way suitable to Fatima. With this freedom bestowed on her, Fatima was able to generously offer a few days a week to act in her loving grandmotherly role while knowing that she had the other days for herself, to explore and grow in areas that appealed to her.

The Health Care Professional's Point of View

The experience of Fatima, Angela, and Frank is a perfect example of wrong assumptions that may lead to family strife and, in this case, an almost pathological emotional state on the part of one member of the family. Almost any family situation can result in misunderstandings, and if they aren't addressed in an open and honest way, they can lead to family dysfunction. There are many families in which misunderstandings or crossed communications have led to disruptions that last for many years and, if not dealt with, become irreversible.

Sometimes stereotyping or traditional gender-based roles may interfere with family members fulfilling their personal goals and expectations. Many older women recall their childhood experiences when they were directed to choose a career path or personal direction based on assumptions of what was "right" for a girl. Of course nowadays, that is less common and most mature women feel they have the right and personal obligation to fulfill their own interests and aspirations. We may forget, however, that our parents may feel the same way as us, even though they never have had the chance to act that way in the past.

> *Most mature women feel they have the right and personal obligation to fulfill their own interests and aspirations. We may forget, however, that our parents may feel the same way as us, even though they may never have had the chance to act that way in the past.*

An important key to mature and respectful relationships is open and honest communication. When we feel thwarted or unable to address an important personal issue because of fear of rejection or anger or disappointment, we may turn in to ourselves and develop the kind of symptoms that Fatima manifested, in this case what appeared to be a depressive state. She felt "trapped" by the assumptions made by her daughter and her own true devotion to her child and her grandchildren. She was even willing to make the personal sacrifice of not addressing the issue with her daughter, but her deep emotional strife manifested itself in her behaviour. It is fortunate that Angela, being a caring and sensitive daughter, sought to help her mother without realizing the source of her emotional problem.

Fatima did not have the courage or perhaps the practice of expressing her own wishes or needs and accepted the situation rather than "disappoint" her daughter. This is where a knowledgeable and sensitive physician can play a crucial role in helping solve a family problem. The trust that most people feel toward their doctor allows the physician to use his or her experience and knowledge to influence the decisions that families may make. In this case, giving the opportunity for Fatima to express herself privately to the doctor, away from her daughter, was key to figuring out what was going on. All older patients, when visiting a doctor, especially a new one, should have the opportunity to speak to the doctor alone and in confidence, if they are able to do so. Many doctors structure their interview to include all family members during the initial history taking and then provide a chance to examine the patient alone, thereby allowing the person to express his or her own feelings in private. Doctors should try and structure their visits to accommodate this need to be able to speak to the patient privately and confidentially.

Once the issue is recognized it is important to discuss it with everyone involved, and here again the physician can play a role in helping the different players in the situation understand that there is no "blame" involved but rather a misunderstanding of what went into making the decision. In this case, Angela's response was most crucial. Had she berated her mother for not being a caring parent and grandparent, or made her feel guilty by saying she decided to go back to work based on Fatima looking after the infant, Fatima may have changed her mind, acquiesced, and then been resentful for many years to come.

This situation worked out well because of Angela's willingness to be open and respectful and the physician's insight into discerning that there was something wrong that did not fit into the usual picture of a true clinical depression. The result is likely to be fruitful and satisfying for everyone with the possibility of Fatima expanding her free days or contracting them, depending on which of her activities gives her the most satisfaction. Or, she may continue with the same mix of time, thereby giving her joy from her family and from her own new achievements and personal growth.

Chapter Five

Culture Clash:
Pitting Values against Needs

When hard, pragmatic decisions are required, differing views and values of parents, their children, and those who influence them can lead to new challenges when trying to decide on the "right" thing to do.

The Challenge

Moshe and Miriam Greenberg were born in Poland. They were teenagers when they met in Warsaw, and both they and their families became very good friends. When the Nazis invaded their country, Moshe was 21 and Miriam had just turned 19.

As Poland crumbled under the onslaught of the German's massive war machine, both Moshe and Miriam's families wanted to flee, but by then the options were few and far between. Trapped, as were hundreds of thousands of other Jewish families, they tried to live their lives as normally as possible. However, that didn't last long at all.

For the first year of German occupation, Moshe and Miriam and their families remained in their homes, although day by day their world kept deteriorating until it was shattered completely when the Nazis announced they would be "moved." That move, of course, was to a concentration camp. Two days before they were herded into trucks, Moshe and Miriam were married in a secret ceremony because they wanted to be together forever—whatever "forever" would come to mean for them.

What followed was almost five years of unimaginable personal terror and horror for each of them. They watched in anguish and anger as family members and friends died before their eyes, or simply vanished, never to be seen again. Sometimes, Moshe and Miriam didn't know for weeks on end whether the other was even alive. But because they were young and in good health at the outset, and because they both had a fierce will to live, at war's end both were still alive—barely. It was weeks after their camp had been liberated that Moshe and Miriam were reunited, both of them mentally and physically scarred.

They slowly recovered their health, and once the emotional pain had subsided to a manageable level, Moshe and Miriam knew they had to get on with rebuilding their world, which was now empty of all their families and most of their friends. Fortunately, Moshe had a cousin who lived in Montreal who sponsored them to come to Canada.

Moshe and Miriam adjusted to their new world with remarkable agility. Thanks to some helping hands and their own sense of drive and purpose, the young couple soon had good entry-level jobs: Moshe learned the tool and die business while Miriam, who had a special skill with numbers, learned to be a bookkeeper in a small textile company.

They worked hard, saved money as they could, and forged ahead. In 1952 they bought a small house on the outskirts of the city, and a year later Miriam gave birth to their first child, a son they named Seth. Two years later, she had another son, Isaac. Helen was born 18 months later.

As the years moved on, the Greenberg family remained very close-knit. Moshe and Miriam were very traditional in their religious beliefs and practices, and carefully and thoughtfully observed all the Jewish holidays. Moshe took his sons to synagogue every Friday night and often talked to them about the importance of their heritage and the huge pains inflicted on their family and their people during the course of history, and especially during the past world war.

Eventually, Moshe and Miriam's children reached adulthood and each went off in search of their own destinies. Seth became a chartered accountant and landed a good job with a Toronto-based firm specializing in the lucrative field of forensic accounting. Isaac, who had always loved music and was an accomplished pianist, studied business in university and ended up managing a number of rock groups, bands, and singers. Helen studied physiotherapy and started a small but successful clinic with three partners that grew into a real going concern.

As the children moved ahead with their own lives, Moshe noted that Seth, Isaac, and Helen and their families spent less and less time with their parents, and they seemed to drift away from the strong religious grounding he and Miriam had instilled.

Several years ago, Moshe and Miriam moved into a retirement home that had an adjacent long-term nursing facility. They continued to live fairly independently, with daily support services. Their three children and their spouses and grandchildren visited regularly and phoned often to check on them and discuss their needs.

Now, Moshe is 82 years old. His health has been steadily failing the past five years. First, he was diagnosed as a diabetic. A year later, he suffered a mild heart attack that left him weakened and more tentative because he was afraid of another more severe attack. But instead of another heart attack, Moshe suffered a stroke, and then another. Since his second stroke, Moshe has been unable to speak or move his left arm or leg. He's lost control of his bowels and has having a very difficult time chewing his food. Late last year, Moshe was transferred to the long-term nursing facility, while Miriam moved to a smaller apartment in the retirement home.

At 80, Miriam is still vigorous and mentally alert. She visits her husband at least twice a day and sometimes sits with him for several hours at a time.

Seth, Isaac, and Helen have discussed their father's health, acknowledging that he is on a course of steady deterioration. They have talked with their mother about the future, urging her to consider allowing him to pass on if there are any further complications.

Miriam was very upset about her children's suggestion and turned to her rabbi for advice. Rabbi Rubinfeld was very clear and firm in his counsel to her: the sanctity of life is more important than any other factor, he told her. He said that was true in Judaism and every other religion, and that no matter what, every effort must always be made—with no exceptions—to keep any living being alive. Miriam accepted his wisdom totally and told her children about how she felt.

What her children saw, though, was a father who was a shell of the man they knew and whose life was barely livable. But their mother made it clear that she was in charge of the situation, and that as long as she was of sound mind her first priority was to keep her husband alive. Besides, she told them, not only were there new medicines and treatments coming on the market almost every day, she knew that people in their father's condition did improve sometimes, so that couldn't be ruled out either.

In what they thought might be a good step to take, Seth, Isaac, and Helen decided that Seth should meet with Rabbi Rubinfeld and ask for his support. Seth explained to the rabbi that he and his brother and sister were worried about their father's quality of life, and he asked the rabbi to help prepare their mother for a difficult decision that was bound to have to be made sometime. The rabbi, however, was steadfast and told Seth that he couldn't help, given his own strong convictions.

Meanwhile, Moshe contracted pneumonia and required treatment with antibiotics and oxygen, but he recovered. However, it was clear to the physicians and nurses that the reason he contracted pneumonia was because of the difficulty he has swallowing. They felt that he would need a feeding tube to provide nourishment and fluids to maintain him and to reduce the risk of further episodes of pneumonia. The doctor at the nursing home asked Miriam what she would like to do. He said they could try feeding him again, but that if he developed another bout of pneumonia he could die from it. On the other hand, the feeding tube had some risks, although for the most part was a fairly safe procedure.

The doctor also explained the situation to Seth when he came to check on his father. Seth called his sister and brother to tell them about the choice they had to make. One of the nurses caring for Moshe indicated to Seth in private that she thought it would be cruel to prolong their father's "suffering" by putting in a tube and that she could never understand families that made that decision.

On a different occasion two nurses spoke to Helen and said that Miriam was so devoted that even with a tube her father could still have some meaningful and comfortable life ahead of him.

The three siblings then arranged to visit their mother, and they pleaded with her to let events take their course without putting in a feeding tube, which they felt would just prolong their father's suffering. Only Helen was ambivalent about not feeding her father—not so much for religious reasons, but because of the idea of "starving" him, especially with her knowledge of the symbolic meaning of food for her parents because of the Holocaust experience. Seth and Isaac told their mother that while they loved their father, watching him like this was very painful for them and they wondered if he would have wanted a feeding tube had he been able to make such a decision himself. They felt he would not.

Miriam was furious. She told Seth and Isaac that she felt they were betraying their father and their faith. She appealed to Helen for support. She said that since she was the decision-maker she simply wouldn't talk about it any more because she believed Moshe, as an observant Jew, would follow Rabbi Rubinfeld's advice about the feeding tube. She reminded them of the terrible ordeal she and Moshe had experienced so many years ago, and said that was evidence that one should never, ever give up on living.

> *Miriam was furious. She told Seth and Isaac that she felt they were betraying their father and their faith.*

Now, there is a high level of tension between Seth, Isaac, and their mother, with Helen not quite sure if her mother is right in making this decision. They would like the rabbi to be more "realistic" in the advice he is giving to their mother.

The Health Professional's Point of View

Conflicts over cultural, ethnic, and religious perspectives are common in any multicultural society. In the health care profession, we usually think of the conflict as being one in which a patient and family have their own peculiar perspective which is not understood or shared by the health care team, thereby leading to unnecessary conflicts. In fact, many health care organizations and health care professionals attempt to find ways to get advice about and assistance to help them with cultures they do not fully understand.

There are always cases where the health care staff, because of a failure to understand and appreciate the underlying values and beliefs that determines a family's decision, end up in situations of terrible conflict. There are even cases that have made their way through the court system because, for example, a family's belief in the sanctity of life persuaded them to demand that the patient be kept on a respirator following a severe motor vehicle accident, even though the health care team felt that the there was no chance of a good recovery and that it was a "waste" to continue with intensive care treatments. In other cases, some health care team members might be so intent on allowing the patient to have the final say that they fail to recognize and appreciate that in a particular culture, it is the accepted practice for the eldest son to make a decision and "protect" the parent from the pain associated with such a step.

All religious, cultural, and ethnic groups have beliefs and rituals with special meaning and importance to those who follow the tenets of the particular group involved. It is important for health care providers to understand where decisions come from so that they can best support the decision-makers.

In this particular case, the problem appears to be an estrangement of underlying values between Miriam and at least two of her children, coupled with different health care team members providing conflicting advice to family members. It is often the case that different generations with different life experiences have incongruent value systems when facing difficult end-of-life situations. As for the staff, they should not be providing advice based on their own personal values to a family in turmoil. Rather, they should limit their advice to the factual level of whether feeding tubes could safely provide nourishment to Moshe and decrease the risk of aspiration pneumonia.

> *It is often the case that different generations with different life experiences have incongruent value systems when facing difficult end-of-life situations.*

What is the best way to support this family and do everything possible to help them through a difficult period so that after Moshe dies they will still be a loving and caring family?

First of all, the children have to accept that their mother is the rightful surrogate decision-maker, whether they agree with her values or not, and that she appears to be acting in a way that is consistent with Moshe's religious beliefs. From their past actions, it is clear that Miriam and Moshe have taken pride in their Judaism and expressed a commitment to follow its tenets. This would mean for most observant Jews, that when there is a difficult situation and a rabbi's advice is sought, that advice must be followed.

For Miriam, the concept of sanctity of life is very important and that was emphasized to her by the rabbi she consulted. He also would have told her that providing food is an obligation except when doing so itself causes harm, and so giving Moshe a feeding tube would be an extension of that obligation to feed.

If Moshe was not likely to survive the pneumonia and was in fact dying, the rabbi might very well have given different advice to Miriam. For most religious Jews, the obligations concerning the care of a dying person are different and comfort becomes paramount, so a feeding tube might not be inserted. For Miriam, it is clear that the religious rules and obligations were important to her husband, as they are to her. She would likely take great comfort after Moshe dies knowing that she assured his care was in the religious tradition of Judaism, even if the outcome was not what she wanted. If on the other hand, she were to ignore what she would interpret as his wishes, she would likely carry the guilt with her for the rest of her life and blame herself for not doing the "right thing."

The children, who are no longer committed to Jewish tradition and law (known as Halacha), may fail to appreciate that certain rules exist which may not make sense to them in a secular world. Similar value systems are shared by Muslims and for many of the Catholic faith. On the other hand, people from Southeast Asia may approach the same situation differently from someone from South America and still differently from someone from the Caribbean.

Seth and Isaac may have difficulty understanding why Miriam is so intent on trying to keep their father alive when he appears to have such a poor quality of life. Helen appears to be in a better position to support her mother's wishes whatever they may be, and that will be very important for Miriam as she struggles through this difficult period. It is terrible to feel alone when making difficult decisions, and children are often key to being able to survive emotionally during trying situations.

It might be worthwhile for Seth and Isaac, if they have forgotten the basic tenets of Judaism when it comes to decisions such as these, to meet with the rabbi privately for an explanation of the basis of the decision. Even if they long ago abandoned their own Jewish religious beliefs, they are likely able to project sufficiently to understand the basic underpinnings of the faith and how it affects decisions. If they could successfully bring themselves to see the situation from their mother's perspective, they could likely be a great support to her. Even if in their own hearts Seth and Isaac disagree with the decision, if they can accept that it is consistent with their parents' belief system and embrace it and its possible consequences (i.e., Moshe being kept alive for a period of time with a feeding tube in place), it would go a long way to restoring family peace.

For families in which the value-based ties have been splintered, it is important for children to step back a bit and try to imagine the values of their parents. By doing this, they should be able to understand how important it may be for them to follow through in the practice of the religion or culture that they hold. Many people who appear to have abandoned their religion during their adult years find comfort in the traditions and practices as they approach death. There is nothing inconsistent or hypocritical in this shift, and everything should be done to support people who need to revert to previously held beliefs, even those they may have ignored for years, if that is what appears to make them comfortable during their remaining days.

Seth, Isaac, and Helen should try and find a way to gather around Miriam and tell her that whatever decision she makes is the right one and that they understand the Judaic reasons for the decision and support her in that difficult choice.

If Moshe lives for many months, even if he does not improve at all, they must not waiver in their support of her decision. If on the other hand, a tube is inserted and Moshe succumbs, they can feel comfort in the fact that they supported their mother's decision to do the "right thing" according to Judaism. That support will give her comfort for the days, months, and years ahead when she thinks about what transpired during those terrible days of Moshe's last illness.

Chapter Six

Substance Abuse:
Drinking All Day Keeps Reality Away

PARENTS WHO ARE UNWILLING OR UNABLE TO cope with their lives sometimes resort to excessive drinking, or taking too many medications. It is especially dangerous if drugs and alcohol are mixed, which can lead to dire consequences and to huge concerns for the children.

The Challenge

Gilles Ducet is a 78-year-old widower who lives in a small two-bedroom home in Trois Rivières, Quebec. Gilles was a construction worker from the time he left school when he was 17 until he retired at age 66. Over the years, Gilles worked hard; he was physically strong because of the type of work he did. He always liked to have his few beers with his buddies at the end of the day, followed by several shots of whiskey in the evenings after dinner. When Gilles retired, he kept drinking but began putting on weight because he wasn't nearly as physically active.

His wife, Hélène, died six years ago of cancer. They were very close and her death was a terrible blow for Gilles. He retreated into his house, and further into himself, for several years. And he drank more, although he denied it to his twin 52-year-old daughters, Eva and Estelle.

Two years ago, Gilles was in a minor car accident late one night, and he was charged with impaired driving. His licence was suspended, and although he can now reapply for a licence, he never has. The fact is that Gilles rarely leaves his house since the accident; the most he does outdoors is mow his small lawn in the summer and sweep the snow if it's not too deep during the long winter months.

Estelle, who is divorced and alone, lives and works as a real estate broker in Trois Rivières. She visits her father once a week for an hour or two, but because she often finds him tipsy, argumentative, and moody, she rarely enjoys the visits.

Eva lives in Montreal with her second husband; they have no children and are financially secure, which in their case means they often enjoy travelling to distant destinations for several weeks at a time. Eva visits her father about once a month and calls weekly, although like her sister, she doesn't derive much pleasure or satisfaction from the encounters.

About a year ago, Gilles met and became friends with Claudia, a widow who is 10 years younger than Gilles and who lives in a nearby apartment. Claudia now spends most of her time with Gilles at his home.

In comparing notes, Estelle and Eva agree that Claudia seems to tolerate their father's drinking. In fact, they believe Gilles gives Claudia money to buy his beer and whiskey. They also find that Claudia is not particularly open or friendly with either of them, and she usually defends Gilles in any discussion about his lifestyle or drinking. As worrisome to the daughters, they believe that their father is lavishing gifts on Claudia, and that Claudia is under the misguided impression that despite his meagre lifestyle, Gilles has a lot of money.

Both Estelle and Eva have noticed over the past few months that their father's tolerance for whiskey has declined, but not his consumption.

Both Estelle and Eva have noticed over the past few months that their father's tolerance for whiskey has declined, but not his consumption. This, of course, results in his being inebriated most of the time. And recently, Estelle discovered that her father is also taking tranquilizers prescribed by his doctor.

Although she didn't like doing it, Estelle called the doctor to ask him about the tranquilizers and whether he knew about Gilles's drinking. The doctor acknowledged that he knew Gilles was an occasional drinker, but not that he drank as much as Estelle claimed. The doctor also confided that he gave Gilles the prescription because at his last visit Gilles said he was still very depressed about Hélène's death and about his own deteriorating condition. It was clear to Estelle from this conversation that Gilles has never talked to his doctor about his drinking and that the doctor hasn't picked up on the problem.

Estelle then called Eva, and the two of them went to visit their father. They confronted him about the drinking, but he denied that he drank too much and was very defensive. They also told him that they were worried about what to them appeared to be memory lapses and poor judgment during recent visits and telephone calls, and they wondered if mixing the liquor with the tranquilizers was wreaking havoc on his mind and body. If anything, they told their father, he seemed more depressed than ever.

Gilles was adamant in his rebuttal of his daughters' allegations and dismissed their concerns. He got quite angry and told them that his life was much better now that Claudia was part of it, how she looked after him with much more care and attention than his own daughters, and how much that meant to him. Then he told them that he'd asked Claudia to move in with him. They would both benefit, their father explained, because Gilles would always have someone around, and Claudia would be able to save the money she paid for her apartment. It was at this point in their heated exchange that Claudia arrived, and a strained, polite, and inconsequential conversation followed before Estelle and Eva left.

The sisters both went home. Later that night they had a long telephone debate about what to do and how to do it. They agreed that most worrisome for them was Claudia's move into the house with their father. Not only didn't they particularly like or trust Claudia, more importantly they felt certain the woman would continue to supply their father with all the beer and whiskey he wanted. In addition, they feared Claudia had a self-serving agenda: to save her own money and live off Gilles's limited savings.

The more Eva and Estelle talked, the more other fears surfaced, like the thought that Claudia would somehow manipulate their father into assigning ownership of the house to her, or talking him into giving her power of attorney and then having him institutionalized, selling the house, and walking away with what was left of his modest savings. They also worried about their father's failing health and mental capacity, but they didn't know what to do next because they weren't sure Gilles's doctor was paying close enough attention to the real needs of his patient.

The Health Care Professional's Point of View

This is a difficult situation for Gilles's daughters. They should have many concerns, the first being the psychological and physical well-being of their father.

Gilles is on a path to almost certain severe consequences of consuming excessive alcohol combined with tranquilizers. The risk is twofold: first is the negative effect of alcohol on his neurological function and the potentially serious damage to other organs such as his liver, and second is the effect of his depression on his health. Alcohol and tranquilizers aggravate depression, and if no intervention takes place, Gilles is also at risk for doing something serious such as committing suicide. Older men have a very high suicide rate and when they decide on the act they often succeed, using rather violent methods such as hanging or guns. If Gilles is indeed depressed over his wife's death, he might benefit from medical treatment of a combination of antidepressant medication coupled with counselling or psychotherapy.

Another confounding aspect to this situation is the role of Claudia. The children may be suspicious of her intentions, but she may, in fact, have true affection for Gilles with no ulterior motives. Whatever the situation, the daughters will likely require her co-operation in their attempt to help their father. If they find that she is an obstacle to his well-being, the situation is more complex and may require some legal action to protect their father.

Assuming that Claudia cares for Gilles but does not realize the risks of his drinking and use of tranquilizers, Estelle and Eva must discuss the situation with her. They will need Claudia's assistance to achieve their goals of getting Gilles to stop drinking and taking tranquilizers, and of getting proper treatment for his depression. They will also need the assistance of Gilles's family physician, with whom they should have a meeting.

The sequence of meetings depends on whether Claudia is in agreement with them about Gilles's condition or is part of the problem. If Claudia proves to be an ally, she might join them when they meet with the doctor. Or she might prefer to defer to the daughters to outline the situation to the doctor and confirm that she is willing to co-operate in any fashion required to assist Gilles, for whom she cares a lot.

At the meeting with the doctor, the daughters must impress upon him that they are observing serious changes in their father's mood and cognitive function. They must use words and examples that describe sufficiently their observations so that the doctor can understand that Gilles is doing his best to hide the extent of his drinking and is not adequately expressing the degree of his depression. If the physician agrees to assist Estelle and Eva, an appointment should be made for Gilles to see the doctor. This can be arranged either by the daughters or at the initiation of the doctor.

The daughters should explain to Gilles that they have concerns about his drinking and that they really believe a visit to the doctor would be helpful. If he refuses, the doctor might be able to assist by calling Gilles and asking him to visit to make sure that he is all right. Subterfuge in such situations does not usually work because the whole process should be based on trust, and if Gilles begins to not trust his daughters' devotion to him, it will be very hard to resolve this complex situation.

If Gilles agrees to visit his physician and if Claudia agrees with and supports the goal of decreasing Gilles' alcohol consumption, then Claudia should accompany the daughters on the visit. Then, together, they can express their love and devotion to Gilles and their desire to help him.

The physician can be extremely helpful in how he approaches Gilles's drinking problem. It is well known that people who abuse alcohol and other drugs that effect mood usually deny their problem. An approach by the physician that is non-judgmental but that rather focuses on the effects on Gilles's mental function is likely to have the best impact. People like Gilles are more likely to listen to a straightforward explanation that continuous exposure of the brain to alcohol can lead to a condition of dementia similar to Alzheimer's disease. Few people are willing to risk the loss of their cognitive function when the implications are laid out (e.g., loss of independence, loss of memory and judgment, inability to simple tasks such as dressing and going to the toilet). A discussion about the negative effect on sexual function may also be effective. Gilles may already be aware of this phenomenon and not realize the connection to alcohol use. This discussion should include the potential benefits of using a proper combined therapy for depression with antidepressant medication and counselling.

One visit alone to the doctor may not be sufficient. The physician should be willing to initiate a process by which to assist Gilles in the very challenging process of recognizing that there is a problem and then taking the steps to address it. The physician might suggest counselling from a social worker or psychologist if there is someone with that expertise available. There may be a special program in the community available for people dealing with substance abuse (the term often used for excessive use of alcohol and medications that effect the brain's function). If so, a recommendation to access the services might be part of what the physician suggests.

> *The most important part of the process is a commitment to help Gilles even if he does not follow through exactly as everyone would like.*

The most important part of the process is a commitment to help Gilles even if he does not follow through exactly as everyone would like. Sometimes an agreement to gradually cut back on the amount of alcohol consumed is a reasonable first step. This type of arrangement is important to consider because alcohol abusers usually can't imagine completely discontinuing their drinking. Also there is a potential danger of seizures occurring, which can happen when alcohol is suddenly discontinued, and which can be very frightening and sometimes cause serious injury. So a gradual approach with the support of everyone who cares for Gilles is necessary to achieve the goal.

If things go well, Gilles will gradually decrease his alcohol intake and the tranquilizers will be discontinued. At some point a decision will likely be made to undertake treatment with antidepressants. It is preferable to discontinue using alcohol before starting these drugs, but sometimes if small doses are started and the results carefully monitored, antidepressants can be introduced while alcohol intake is reduced. Sometimes the antidepressant therapy improves the patient's mental state so that the commitment to stop drinking becomes stronger and is more readily implemented.

If these steps are followed through, there is a good chance that Gilles can cease his alcohol abuse and respond properly to antidepressant therapy. He can then have a full relationship with his daughters and, if it proves appropriate, with Claudia.

If the situation proves to be more difficult – with Gilles denying there is a problem and Claudia ignoring the concerns of his daughters — the approach is more complex and may require legal intervention. If Claudia is acting in a malicious manner and taking advantage of Gilles, then Eva and Estelle are faced with finding a way to have her effect on Gilles diminished or removed altogether. This will not be easy and may result in Gilles and his daughters becoming alienated. But, if Eva and Estelle are convinced that no alternative is possible, they may have to pursue a legally based course of action. If this is necessary, Gilles may not be amenable to the course of action that is best for him in terms of his alcohol use.

The last option for Estelle and Eva is to let things go and not do anything until some crisis occurs, which may allow them to intervene without causing an affront to Gilles. Such a crisis might be a severe medical consequence of his drinking, such as bleeding from his stomach, a seizure, or severe loss of mental competence which forces decision-making upon the daughters. This is not the way anyone would want the situation resolved, but it may be the only viable option to avoid severe alienation and disruption of the family's fabric and integrity.

Chapter Seven

Siblings:
In Charge and On the Attack

When brothers and sisters vie for attention and favour from an elderly parent, the inevitable outcome is sibling rivalry and mutual distrust. If ever there is a time for siblings to pull together, it's when a parent is in failing health.

The Challenge

Edna Delaney lives in a retirement home in Vancouver. She's a vigorous, high-energy 86-year-old, but she is showing early signs of dementia that is likely Alzheimer's disease, according to her doctor. She's been highly independent since the death of her husband, Frank. From the time he suffered a massive heart attack, Edna blossomed in terms of managing his care and their family finances. Three years after his heart attack, and after steadily declining health, Frank died. Edna grieved greatly, and then seemed to put Frank's death behind her—but not her ongoing love of him—and decided she wanted to live what was left of her life to the fullest.

Edna has four children: Frank Jr., a lawyer who specializes in estate planning who is 57 years old and lives with his family in nearby Burnaby; Joan, 53, a housewife who lives with her family in Victoria; Roger, 51, divorced and living in Los Angeles where he works as an on-again, off-again scriptwriter for various television shows; and Heather, 50, who lives with her second husband and their three children in Ottawa, where she sells real estate.

When their father died, there was some discussion among the four siblings of to best way to help their mother. Given the distances, it was agreed Frank Jr. and Joan would take lead roles, since they were in closest proximity to their mother. Both Roger and Heather pledged to help as needed.

About six months after his father was buried, Frank Jr. talked with his mother about what help she felt she really needed, and what other help she wanted. In that discussion, Edna made it clear that she wanted to remain as independent as possible and not rely on her children. However, she also made it clear that she wanted to stay in touch with them on a regular basis. She said she favoured none over the other, and that she felt that they were all equal in terms of her affection and attention.

Financially, Edna is in extremely good condition. Her husband was very successful in real estate and in the stock market, and Edna's net worth is somewhere in the area of $3.5 million. The greater concern— at least on the surface—is her health and well-being.

All four Delaney children have a pretty good idea of their mother's financial worth. Frank Jr. has a high income that he's invested wisely, and he is the least concerned about what any possible inheritance would mean. Roger, in contrast, is the most financially insecure because his work is sporadic while his lifestyle is pretty expensive, and he's very aware of what a good inheritance could do for his life.

During the past year, Edna has become increasingly confused, uncertain, and forgetful. She's fallen several times in her apartment, laying on the floor until either the maid service found her or until it was noticed in the dining room that she wasn't present for a meal. Although she has been given a panic button to wear around her neck to use in precisely such situations, Edna—either in her stubborn wish for independence or because of her forgetfulness—more often than not chooses to leave the button in her night table drawer.

Due to these experiences, the administrator at Edna's retirement home called Frank Jr. a few weeks ago and explained that his mother required more attention than the home could offer. He suggested that Frank consider how to ensure she gets the level of attention that she seems to increasingly need. They discussed increasing the care provided on-site with some in-home supplementary services, or even a move to a nursing home, which they both believe she would strongly resist.

In addition, a few weeks ago during Edna's annual physical examination, her doctor surmised, based on her movements and a slight tilt to one side, that she may have had a mild stroke The doctor has her scheduled for a CAT scan to see if there is any evidence to support the observations. But the doctor did tell Edna—and also called Frank Jr. to advise him—that there could be other smaller strokes, and that there is a potential for a more serious stroke occurring because of Edna's weight, eating habits, and past history of heavy smoking.

Frank Jr. has shared this information with his brother and sisters. They all agreed at the time that he should take the lead in ensuring their mother has the care that she needs. Based on this collective decision, Frank Jr. has decided that his mother needs more in-home help. He has arranged for her to be moved to a larger apartment in the retirement home and has hired a caregiver, with backup support. In all, Edna's accommodation, meals, and care are now costing nearly $7,000 a month.

Edna has been prescribed medications to improve her function and decrease the likelihood of further strokes, and Frank Jr. has arranged for the pills to be dispensed in a way that Edna will more likely take them correctly. The increase in help is more of an imperative now that her medication regimen is more complex and her care needs are increasing.

Roger, who seldom called or visited his mother in the past, now calls his mother every other day. He has visited her twice in the past six months. Edna confides to Frank Jr. that Roger has suggested that she should move to California to be near him. Roger has also impressed on his mother that the weather there would be better for her. Plus, in all his calls, Roger has probed about her will—again, something Edna tells Frank Jr.—and has urged her to consider which of her children needs and deserves more of her money when she passes away.

Frank Jr., having reflecting on all he's been told and has learned, urges his mother to think through what she wants to do with her will, which hasn't been revised since before her husband died. But he's reluctant to give advice. Despite his vocation, it's an uncomfortable situation for Frank Jr. since this isn't just a client—it's his mother. Heather, in her weekly telephone call, urges her mother to write a new will and plan her life to suit her own level of comfort and needs, pointing out that all her children are adults and can and should look after themselves without any longer depending on her. Finally, Joan, who visits her mother once a month, is subtly lobbying her mother by reminding Edna that she's always there for her, and that she comes to see her regularly.

When Frank Jr. conducts a mental inventory of the state of the family affairs, he realizes that none of Edna's children are really talking to each other about the situation and how to best manage it. He's troubled by this, but not quite certain what to do about it. While busy with his day-to-day work and thinking about how to talk with his mother, Roger arrives for another visit. During that weekend, Roger applies great pressure on Edna to move to Los Angeles and to give him power of attorney over her financial affairs and her health needs. He vows to look after her, telling his mother that that he's the only one who doesn't have family to support and, therefore, he can devote his time and attention to her well-being.

Edna tells Frank Jr. about Roger's thoughtful suggestion. But she's already confused, and when Frank Jr. tells her to think about what's best for her, she confides that Roger made it clear that he was the one who could care for her best, and that the American health care system would do more for her.

A week later, Roger calls his brother and sisters and makes his case for being the prime caregiver and why their mother should move to Los Angeles. He's adamant in his position and pleads for support. Heather is concerned, worried that Roger has an agenda that is self-serving. Joan doesn't know what to think, except that Roger is going to end up with a lot of money. And Frank Jr. is worried that his mother will give in to the pressure being exerted by Roger. None of the siblings feels comfortable with each other or with the way things are shaping up. Nor do any of them know what to do, or how to do it, except for Roger, who the others believe has a clear agenda. Suddenly, there is growing doubt and concern among them and a sense that perhaps they must jockey for their mother's attention and favour.

> *Suddenly, there is growing doubt and concern among the siblings and a sense that perhaps they must jockey for their mother's attention and favour.*

The Health Care Professional's Point of View

The primary focus of all of these deliberations must be Edna. If any of the children forgets this, there must be a way of reminding them clearly, while things are still reasonably stable and before there is a crisis in Edna's care needs or a breakdown in the relationship of the siblings. This may require a family meeting, even if it means that all of them have to visit Vancouver. If that is impossible, they should plan a conference call in which they all can participate. If their basic relationship prior to Edna's decline has been good, this can be built upon to take the steps that will assure Edna's well-being for the present and the future.

There are a number of issues that must be aired during the family discussion. With the necessary information from the doctor (a family meeting with the doctor could be of great value, but might not be logistically possible), it should be possible to get a prognosis and likely timeline of the progression of Edna's medical condition.

If she has Alzheimer's disease as well as suffering from some small strokes, it is pretty clear that there will be continued deterioration of her mental and intellectual functioning. This is the case even if she is considered a suitable candidate for one of the new drugs now used in combatting Alzheimer's disease (e.g., Aricept®, Exelon®, or Reminyl®) which might decrease the rate of decline but will not offer anything like a "cure" for her condition.

With the knowledge that there will be progressive decline, the next question that must be asked is whether, in fact, Edna has the mental capacity to make the kinds of decisions that she is being asked to make, such as changing her will or moving to California. It is likely that if formally tested, she would be found *not* to have the capacity to change her will in any substantive way. If there were changes, these would likely be open to legal challenge after she dies if one of the siblings is not happy with the changes.

If she is not mentally capable of making a new will, it is also unlikely that she can understand and appreciate the implications of a move to California or of making what would be considered a "legally capable decision." Also it should be made clear to all the siblings, especially Roger, that as their mother deteriorates her care needs will increase and she will need a lot of family support, which is unlikely to be available from Roger alone in Los Angeles.

As for the quality of care that Edna may eventually require, she should be able to get as good if not better long-term care at a much lower cost in British Columbia than in Los Angeles. This factor should be considered if there is a concern about her having the funds to sustain her over a long period of decline and perhaps leave a legacy for her children, which seems to be her wish.

With these factors taken into consideration, the discussion of the siblings should include who is going to be the formal spokesperson for the family so that decisions about her health can be made. Unless they agree to a spokesperson to represent them (with, of course, reasonable consultation among themselves), they could end up in a situation in which the courts appoint a guardian in the absence of a defined decision-maker.

> *With these factors taken into consideration, the discussion of the siblings should include who is going to be the formal spokesperson for the family so that decisions about her health can be made.*

Assuming, as most families do, that it is better for them to find a way to co-operate than having an outside person make decisions without their consultation, they will eventually agree to a way by which one of them, likely Frank Jr., is the designated decision-maker (surrogate). It would have been better if prior to Edna losing her capacity that she and her children had discussed the possibilities for the future should she become ill. At that time they could have agreed on this process and structure, rather than leaving it open to potential conflict that may result in resentment among the children as Edna deteriorates.

Assuming that, after hearing the facts and the implications of the various options, the children agree the best arrangement for Edna is to have her stay in Vancouver with Frank Jr. taking the primary care role, they then need to make some backup arrangements. They should agree that when Frank Jr. needs time to go on vacation or travel on business, someone else will be in Vancouver to assure Edna continues her social visits and outings. If this agreement is in place, then it is possible that Frank Jr. will be able to carry on with the main responsibility. Rather than challenging his role, his siblings should be grateful that they have him as a strong support for Edna and not someone who is likely motivated by a future inheritance.

If the situation is not resolved happily, and Roger or one of the other siblings challenges the status quo, it might be necessary for Frank Jr. to go to court and ask that he be appointed the formal surrogate and power of attorney for Edna's financial and personal needs. It is likely that he would be successful in such a request, but the repercussions in terms of family structure and resentment could be so great that the fabric of the family would be irrevocably destroyed after such a legal process. If the children feel inclined to pursue the matter through legal channels, they would be wise to get some impartial advice on the short- and long-term implications for them, for Edna, and for their family relationships.

If the family agrees to Frank Jr.'s role as primary caregiver, they can all focus on making sure that Edna receives the best possible health care as she continues to decline mentally and physically. This will be provided through the co-operation of a loving and devoted family that do their best to make her comfortable and visit as often as possible, considering that some of the children live far away. Whatever financial legacy might be left to them, the most important legacy is the knowledge that they cared for their mother, taking into account her best interests and not their own.

CHAPTER EIGHT

The Stroke:
Sudden Challenges and Changes

A SELF-SUFFICIENT PARENT SUFFERS A series of strokes, creating an instant family crisis requiring careful co-ordination of care and attention.

The Challenge

Diane is 51 years old and married to Terry, who is 55. They have an 18-year-old daughter, Amanda. This is Terry's second marriage. He divorced his first wife after 15 years of an unhappy and acrimonious marriage that produced a daughter, Jill, who is 23 years old and lives on her own.

Diane's father left her mother, Wilma, more than a decade ago. A quick divorce followed and he's not been heard from since. Diane, while never close to her father or approving of his lifestyle and treatment of her mother, still on occasion wonders about him.

Terry lost both of his parents in a fatal automobile accident six years ago while on their way for a vacation in Florida.

Because both Diane and Terry were the only children in their families, neither of them have any close family to speak of other than a few distant cousins and an uncle out west. That's why they are so close to Diane's mother, Wilma.

Until recently, Wilma lived on her own in a large, rambling house an hour's drive in the country from Diane and Terry's home in Saskatoon. She'd lived there ever since her husband had left her. Wilma had never remarried, but for the past five or six years she has been casually seeing a widower who lived not far from her; they were just good friends (or so it seemed) who enjoyed being together.

Diane often drove out just to visit her mother for an hour or so. As well Diane and Terry regularly visited Wilma, with a protesting Amanda in tow. Not that Amanda didn't like her grandmother; she was just at an age when she would rather spend all her time with her friends and not her parents. However, despite not wanting to go—especially for weekend visits—Amanda usually had a reasonably good time once she got there. And Wilma, who at 72 years of age was full of energy, would take the bus to the city and visit for several days at a time with her daughter and family.

Wilma had always been in good health. The first time in her life that she'd been in the hospital was four years ago for a day surgery cataract procedure. She faithfully went to her annual medical checkups, and she always faired well in the final assessments. Her one big problem was her weight. Wilma loved her food and loved to eat. She was about 50 pounds overweight, and no amount of frequent but loosely applied dieting got her weight down.

On one of her short visits to see her mother, Diane observed that Wilma was talking with a slight slur and that she leaned to one side in a way that she hadn't noticed before. But for all intents and purposes, Wilma seemed to be fine, just as full of energy as ever. However, Diane did ask her mother if she were feeling all right, and Wilma assured her she couldn't be better. Yet something kept nagging at Diane, and she pressured her mother to make an appointment to see her doctor.

Two days later, Diane called her mother in the morning—a time she was always home—and there was no answer. Troubled, she called Wilma's friend, who said he hadn't seen her in a couple of days. After getting no answer a few more times, Diane called one of Wilma's neighbours and asked if she'd look to see if her mother was there. She wasn't.

Worried, Diane cancelled her next two meetings and drove to her mother's house. Just as she arrived, there was Wilma getting out of the local taxi. Wilma explained that she'd been to see her doctor, who wondered if she might have suffered a very small stoke. But, her mother said, everything seemed to be all right, though the doctor did suggest that she needed "a good going over."

And that's how Diane happened to be there when, an hour later, her mother toppled out of her chair, not able to speak or move. Diane managed to help her mother to the car and drove to the small local hospital. Her doctor was summoned. He confirmed she'd had another stroke and that this one was substantial. He arranged to transfer Wilma to the larger regional hospital.

The next two days were a terrible blur for Diane. She was told that her mother had suffered a massive stroke. Wilma's entire right side was immobile, and she initially lost all ability to speak. After the first day, she could communicate, but only with a few halting words. Terry was shaken and Amanda was in tears. Even Jill, who didn't feel a great deal of closeness to Diane's mother, was moved to ask how she might help.

Diane arranged for her mother to be transported to a hospital in the city, where she could get more sophisticated care and diagnostic tests, and where she'd be closer to the family. A week later, Wilma was transferred again—this time to a rehabilitation hospital as a temporary measure. By now, although Wilma could utter a handful of words, it was clear from all the medical advice Diane had managed to collect that her mother probably would never walk again and certainly couldn't live on her own. Wilma was on a regimen of daily therapy sessions, which seemed to help somewhat, but there was no significant improvement. Nor was there any further deterioration in her condition. All in all, Wilma was holding her own, and she was trying to be as co-operative as possible.

Since entering the rehabilitation hospital, Wilma has had yet another stroke, albeit a much smaller one. She is now totally dependent on full-time care and assistance. She can't walk at all, and she has lost all use of her right arm. She is unable to move out of her bed or wheelchair without help. She has also developed some problems with swallowing and eating and occasionally tends to choke on her food. A nutritionist has made some recommendations about positioning her when she eats and setting the pace of feeding as well as modifying the consistency of foods.

Totally unprepared for this devastating event, Diane and Terry wonder what they should do next to help Wilma and make her as

> Totally unprepared for this devastating event, Diane and Terry wonder what they should do next to help Wilma and make her as comfortable as possible.

comfortable as possible. They aren't certain where Wilma could live. They recognize that, even though they have a small guest room in their house, Diane's mother needs a level of attention that they can't provide, and they have no room for a full-time caregiver. They also know they have limited time because of their job pressures, and limited resources because they paid for Amanda to go to a private school and now she attends university in the United States. However, they do want to do the right thing for Wilma.

The Health Care Professional's Point of View

The question that Diane and her family must ask is, "What is the right thing to do?" The main focus of the answer should be deciding where Wilma will get the best care for her immediate and long-term needs and what the family can reasonably be expected to do under their present living circumstances.

While it might be that the ideal situation for Wilma to move in with her family, after they renovate the house to accommodate her and arrange for full-time help, this is not possible for Diane and Terry. It would be a monumental undertaking and also a very expensive one. The cost of 24-hour-a-day care is prohibitive for most families unless they are very well off financially. This is not the situation with Diane and Terry, who are, in fact, struggling with their own financial situation now that their daughter is in university.

If the option of keeping Wilma at home is not viable, the only other choice is to find a suitable long-term care facility. They can look for a facility either near where they live or near Wilma's own home. They need to weigh the importance of Wilma being near her social network of friends and neighbours against the convenience of being nearer to the family, who will be Wilma's main support.

Assuming that Wilma is not able to communicate, it may be necessary for her family to try and explore who among her friends might really be available to visit her. If the only important person is her male friend from her neighbourhood, they might speak to him about how they can arrange for him to visit her from time to time. Perhaps they could either periodically pick him up or arrange for his transportation so that he could spend an afternoon at Wilma's nursing home and make a nice visit out of it. Wilma may or may not be able to recognize or fully interact with her friend, but if they could continue some kind of a meaningful relationship, it is worth pursuing this avenue for her benefit.

The rest of the visiting will be up to the family. Although not easy, they should try to develop some plans that will make each visit a bit special. For example, they might bring some treats that are appropriate for Wilma. Of course, if they bring food, it is important to make sure that it is something that she can eat, especially since she has some swallowing difficulties. If Wilma likes flowers, it may be worth putting some plants in her room, as long as someone will take care of them. Taking pictures to share with Wilma would also be a very nice way to keep her up to date with family events.

Going for a walk around the premises is usually something special for nursing home residents and is generally something staff cannot do frequently. Some families hire private companions once in awhile to take their loved one on an outing or walk depending on the situation. If the staff thinks it is safe, going for a drive or some other kind of outing might also be a nice way to change things and bring something new and special into Wilma's life. If music is something special for her, they should arrange for a CD player or tape machine for her room that she can listen to whenever she wants.

This would also be a very good time for Diane and Terry to explore with Wilma what she would like to happen should things take a turn for the worse. For example, if Wilma has strong views about end-of-life issues based on deep-seated personal or religious reasons, these should be confirmed. If it is thought that she would prefer not to have "heroic" treatments provided, this should be established as reasonably as possible. The issue of feeding tubes might also be considered in view of the problems that Wilma is already experiencing with her eating. These issues can be presented in a way that does not frighten Wilma, but as an assurance that nothing will be done for her or to her that she would not want if she could express her wishes herself.

If effective communication takes place, it may be possible for Diane and Terry to understand reasonably the limits and boundaries of care that Wilma would prefer if she were able to communicate at the time. So, for example, if she gets an infection, she would want to be treated if there was a good chance of full recovery. But she might prefer to not have cardiopulmonary resuscitation in the event of a cardiac arrest, or she may not want a permanent feeding tube should she not be able to again eat normally. Knowing Wilma's wishes now, when Wilma's condition is stable and non-threatening, would certainly make it much easier for Diane and Terry to live with what are often difficult decisions at a time of crisis.

These are not easy times or easy decisions. But with the goodwill and dedication that appear to be motivating Diane and her husband, and with a bit of luck, Wilma should be able to manage reasonably well for some time in the nursing home, perhaps months to years.

These are not easy times or easy decisions. But with the goodwill and dedication that appear to be motivating Diane and her husband, and with a bit of luck, Wilma should be able to manage reasonably well for some time in the nursing home, perhaps months to years. She might even improve in terms of function for a while, but then inevitably something will occur from which she cannot recover. Diane and Terry should be ready for all eventualities and be thankful for any period of comfort and enjoyment that Wilma can experience during this very difficult period of her life.

CHAPTER NINE

Dementia and Depression:
Reading the Signs

DISCOVERING THAT A PARENT HAS SIGNIFICANT HEALTH problems but is in total denial is a disturbing and often frightening experience for children. Such a stressful situation requires careful action to best help all involved.

The Challenge

Al and Denise Wilson have been married for 45 years. Al is 72 years old, and Denise is 68. They've both been in excellent health all their lives.

Al retired at age 65 on a full pension after working with the same company since completing university. At about the same time, Denise opted to take a downsizing severance package at the company where she'd been a secretary for more than 30 years, and this provided her with a good pension also.

Al, a structural engineer with a mid-sized consulting company, was actually relieved to retire when he did. He'd found the last couple of years at the office to be increasingly difficult. What bothered Al was that periodically, sometimes for a number of months at a time, he found he was having a harder time concentrating on his assignments, and the more complex a job was, the longer it took him to complete it. He never mentioned this to anyone, and he told himself it was because he was bored and tired after so many years of doing the same thing. He also had periods when he had problems sleeping, and so attributed his lack of concentration to his periodic lack of sleep. Al also thought part of the problem may be that he was eagerly anticipating retirement.

After considering what they really wanted to do in their golden years, Al and Denise sold their comfortable home in Toronto and moved into a retirement community on the shores of a lake north of the city. The transition, which worried them a bit, went very smoothly. As they're still fond of telling people they meet, they both adjusted "like a duck to water"; they had no second thoughts, and certainly no regrets. They've thoroughly enjoyed their lifestyle in their new home. They cultivated friendships with a number of other retired couples, played bridge weekly, and, best of all, they both golfed every other day. Last year, they splurged and bought a small sailboat and took some lessons. During the summer months they sailed most evenings for an hour on the lake.

The past several years, Al and Denise have spent six weeks each winter in Florida at a condominium they share with another couple they've known for years. All in all, Al and Denise are very much enjoying their lives and feel that the years of work and careful savings are paying off handsomely.

Their only child, Mary, is 37 years old and lives in Toronto with her husband, Bob, and their two children, Amy, who is 17, and Tom, who is 14. Mary and her family are close to her parents and visit them about once every two weeks—sometimes staying for a weekend. Most holidays are spent together. Meanwhile, Bob's parents live in North Bay and both are in good health. Twice a year his parents come to visit them in Toronto, and at least annually they trek to North Bay to visit for a few days. And of course, they all talk to each other on the telephone regularly. For all intents and purposes, all the family members honestly like one another and get along well.

About four months ago, Denise noticed for the first time that Al was "not his old self," as she described it to Mary at the time. He seemed to be more withdrawn, she'd told Mary, and sometimes indecisive about things like what to eat—something about which he'd always had very fixed views with strong likes and dislikes.

Mary forgot about what her mother told her, and Denise herself put it somewhere on the back burner of her mind for the time.

As the weeks passed, Denise realized that her husband was spending less and less time in his small woodworking shop that he'd equipped in part of the garage. Finally, she asked him about it. Al said he'd just lost interest in woodworking: that it was too time consuming and too hard. Yet Denise knew Al truly enjoyed making small pieces of furniture and prided himself on the detailed work. That's why a few days later she asked about his woodworking again, this time to enquire when he'd finally build her the shelves above the washer and dryer.

Al became very agitated. He said he didn't know when he might have the time to build the shelves. When Denise reminded him that he had all the time in the world, Al didn't respond.

So the subject was dropped. Then, just a few weeks later, Al changed his mind about going for their usual after-dinner sail, and did so again a week later. This was definitely not like Al at all, because he loved that little boat and the feel of the breeze on the lake. Denise asked him if something was wrong, and Al said, no, he just didn't feel like sailing these days, as he had some increased pain in his back, the result of an old athletic injury. He claimed that sailing seemed a bit risky for him and that he worries more about their safety out on the water. He seemed even more irritated when she asked again about the shelves. He told her that if she needed the shelves so badly, she should just go out and buy some.

Not long after that conversation, Mary, Bob, Amy, and Tom came for a one-day visit. It was a sunny, warm day and everyone wanted to go sailing, but Al said he didn't feel like it—and that was a first. Mary asked her father several times, but got the same negative response every time.

During the course of the day, Denise pulled her daughter aside and told her about her father's recent change of behaviour and how it was confusing to her. Mary was mystified. She watched her father very closely for the rest of the visit. She noticed that he sometimes appeared withdrawn, as if he was in his own world. He also did not laugh in his usual way at her husband's wisecracks and puns, which was a bit out of character. She mentioned this to her mother later on that evening, who said that this kind of behaviour occurred quite often. Mary asked if there was anything else, and her mother admitted

> *Mary was mystified. She watched her father very closely for the rest of the visit. She noticed that he sometimes appeared withdrawn, as if he was in his own world.*

that Al was no longer interested in sex; whenever she approached him he found an excuse for not participating, usually complaining of fatigue or backache, a problem he had had for years but had never before interfered with what had been, up until a few months ago, a very satisfying sex life for the two of them.

Later Mary told her husband about her observations and comments by her mother, and he suggested that they both must see a doctor for a good assessment.

The next day, Mary called her mother and asked when her parents last had a good medical checkup. Denise became alarmed and wanted to know why Mary was asking. Mary told her mother of her conversation with Bob the night before and reminded her that her father was not himself and withdrawn. She told her mother that there was a lot written lately about depression, especially in older people, and it just seemed like a good idea for both of them to get thorough medical assessments from time to time. Mary told her mother she thought a good assessment would be especially helpful with these changes in her father's behaviour. Denise told Mary that both she and Al had had a good checkup two years ago, but hadn't had any reason to see a doctor since, and that was a blessing.

Still, Mary urged her mother to arrange for medical checkups for both of them. She reminded her mother that just as she, Bob, and the kids get annual checkups, so should her parents. And, Mary argued, it was a matter of something more than a regular routine examination, because it seemed clear that something was not right with her father which had to be identified and addressed.

Later that day Denise sat with Al on their deck, having a glass of wine before dinner. Al lately had started drinking more than a glass before dinner. He said it calmed him down, but Denise didn't think much of it. After all, they were retired and he didn't have to worry about sleeping in if he had an extra drink or two. She suggested that it probably was time for them to both go for a checkup; their doctor was still practising in Toronto, so they could make a day of it—see the doctor, do some shopping, and then come home. Al shot back that he didn't need a medical checkup; he felt just fine, and if she needed one, he'd be pleased to take her. He wouldn't explain why he refused to go, even though Denise asked several times. Finally, Al stated emphatically that he felt just fine, and that there was no use spending time on something that wasn't necessary, and that Denise probably was fine also. He said that they were having the best years of their lives, and that's the way it should be. End of discussion. No matter what approach she took, Denise couldn't get Al to agree to visit the doctor.

A couple of days later, when Mary called to talk with her mother, Denise told her of her father's firm decision, and said she didn't want to provoke him or have an argument about it. So, for the time being, Denise said they would just skip the visit to the doctor and just see how things went, because actually both of them felt well, other than the change in Al's interests and the fact that he seemed to sit around a lot more than usual. And after all, Denise told her daughter, there was really nothing physically wrong with them. Just because Al didn't want to build shelves or sail as often, or wasn't that interested in sex, at least temporarily, it didn't really mean anything. These things happen to people; she figured that it was a "phase" that would pass.

Mary didn't argue or push, feeling that if that's what her parents wanted, that's okay. For all her life, they'd been there for her as solid supporters and sound parents, and she didn't think that the current situation demanded any kind of hard push on her part. She decided that if there were any further visible signs of a problem with her father, she'd personally arrange for and take him to a doctor's appointment. And her mother seemed just fine.

The Health Care Professional's Point of View

It is imperative that Al gets medical advice. It appears from the description that Al is suffering from a depressive illness, which could be occurring for several reasons. In the early stages of dementia, such as Alzheimer's disease, depressive symptoms can be the earliest manifestation, and major depression can occur for the first time in older individuals. Also, sometimes an earlier bout of depression may not have been recognized for what it was, or attributed to "nerves" or "stress" or "overwork" and may have been ignored and not formally treated. A family history of depression sometimes helps with the diagnosis and it would be useful to know if any of Al's siblings or parents ever had problems with mood disorders.

The main obstacle to Al receiving help for depression is either that he is not aware something is wrong or, more likely, he feels ashamed or guilty about admitting that things are "not right." Many older people, especially men who have always been "in charge," have difficulty admitting that things are happening to them that they cannot control. Deep-seated feelings of inadequacy often occur and sexual problems are not uncommon. This just makes things worse, especially if the person is not used to expressing feelings and exploring problems with other people, even his or her spouse.

The danger in depression, especially when it occurs in older men, is that it sometimes leads to suicide. They may not give any real outward warning that things are that bad, but to the surprise of all their loved ones, they kill themselves, often by some violent means. For other men, suicide is not an option, but they withdraw into themselves, eat less, or consume increasing amounts of alcohol and medications such as tranquilizers (that they may get from a doctor after complaining of sleep problems) that temporarily ease their feelings of despair.

A family in this situation needs to find a way to get their loved one to see a physician.... Waiting for something to happen is not the answer. In fact, if they do that and something terrible happens they would never forgive themselves.

A family in this situation needs to find a way to get their loved one to see a physician. Some depressed people will go on their own so that they do not have to involve their family with something of which they may be ashamed. Some people believe that depression is a sign of weakness and they should just be able to "pull themselves out of it." But that rarely happens. So what are Mary and Denise to do?

Waiting for something to happen is not the answer. In fact, if they do that and something terrible happens they would never forgive themselves. It would probably be worthwhile for Mary and Denise to arrange to be alone with Al and have a discussion in which they express their concern for him because of what they have been observing for the past few months. Al's response may be dismissive and he may be angry that they are intruding on his feelings.

It might be helpful for Mary to bring some reading material for Al, suggesting that he read it when he is alone. She and her mother have to express their love and devotion to Al and tell him that they realize just how difficult it might be for him to admit to or express his true feelings. They might suggest that perhaps he would prefer to visit the doctor himself rather than going with Denise. Of course, the hope would be that he declines that offer because they want to be with him when he tells the doctor what has been happening. By himself, he might deny that anything is wrong with his sense of self and value.

Al may not respond immediately to such a conversation. However, reading the material provided by Mary and Denise might provide enough pressure on him so that he agrees to see his doctor. If this is the case, it would be worthwhile communicating with the doctor first by phone or letter to explain the concerns of the family. Then, during the medical assessment, if Al does not admit to any problems, the physician can ask the necessary probing questions that may lead to a diagnosis of depression.

If a diagnosis of depression is made, the likely outcome will be an attempt at treatment with an antidepressant medication. There is a very good chance that the drug will be tolerated, especially if the physician begins with a small dose and gradually increases it, and will also be effective. If so, Al should become more interactive, less withdrawn, and once again become interested in his hobbies and in his wife. Many different antidepressant drugs and other components to treatment including group therapy may be offered, and usually one type of treatment or another will prove successful.

This is a time that a great deal of understanding and support is required, and Denise, Mary, and Bob will have to put all their efforts toward being supportive of Al and giving him the time and space to make his recovery.

One major concern, in addition to the high risk of suicide, is that the depression may be a symptom of dementia. For a substantial percentage of individuals, depressive symptoms respond to treatment, but their mental powers and prowess continue to decline until it becomes clear that something beyond depression is taking place. The earliest signs of Alzheimer's disease are often revealed symptomatically with this kind of pattern.

At present, there are no simple tests that can differentiate true late onset depression from the type that will transform itself into dementia. The positive news is that there are new drugs that many people with Alzheimer's disease appear to benefit from. The medical evidence suggests that even if there is no dramatic improvement in mental and cognitive function, the rate of progress of the disease appears to slow down, giving families and patients a bit more time to live life to its fullest and to make the necessary plans in anticipation of a progressive decline. (This includes taking steps such as appointing a power of attorney and making a will that will withstand external scrutiny or contest.)

So, Mary and Denise need to lovingly get Al to the doctor, relate their observations, and explain their concerns. With a bit of luck, Al will be seen, a diagnosis of depression made, and proper treatment started. And maybe with a little bit of extra luck, Al's condition will not gradually deteriorate until a diagnosis of dementia of the Alzheimer's type is made.

CHAPTER TEN

Advancing Dementia:
When Life Gets More Difficult

WHEN PARENTS ARE DETERIORATING, THEIR CHILDREN must make some hard decisions about how they might best help them be most secure and comfortable, while trying to maintain their own lives and meeting their family commitments.

The Challenge

Dorothy Miller is an 87-year-old widow whose husband, Jack, died three years ago of lung cancer. Dorothy never got over the shock of his death, although Jack had a long period of painful illness. After Jack's funeral, Dorothy remained completely devastated and was often unable to stop crying for several hours at a time.

She continued to live in the one-bedroom apartment in a Moncton seniors' retirement home-style building they'd moved to in the mid-1980s when Jack retired from his job with the railroad. They made the move partially to take some of the strain off their need to care for the house they had been living in and because the seniors' facility offered increased levels of care. After Jack's death, Dorothy went out on her own less and less and depended for personal services more and more on her handful of friends who lived in the same building, as well as from the staff.

Although Dorothy was in relatively good physical condition when Jack died, shortly after she began having a number of complaints about her health. The physician who visited the seniors' home weekly saw Dorothy with increasing frequency. To help her sleep and to "calm her nerves," he prescribed a mild dose of Lorazepam—a tranquilizer. Then six months ago, Dorothy slipped in the lobby of the building, fell backwards pulling her walker with her, and fractured one of her vertebrae. She was in a lot of pain and couldn't get up from the floor on her own. The nurse on duty was summoned, who saw at once that Dorothy was suffering. The staff immediately called for an ambulance and she was taken to the hospital, where she required bed rest and fairly strong painkillers.

According to the doctor at the hospital, Dorothy became quite confused during the first night of her hospitalization, likely from a combination of codeine-containing pain medication and her being in an unfamiliar place. They kept her a few days longer to make sure she settled down, which she did. She was discharged and provided with some home care services including a regimen of physiotherapy to help her get walking again.

Dorothy has one child, Owen, who lives in St. John's, Newfoundland. Owen is 67 years old and has suffered from a degenerative disk condition for more than 15 years; in fact, it's the reason he had to take early retirement from his job piloting fishing vessels. His wife, Louise, is three years his senior and for several decades has suffered from schizophrenia. Her illness is reasonably controlled by medications, but even so, she still has some very difficult times.

Owen and Louise choose to live in St. John's because Louise has supportive family there—two sisters and two brothers and their families, all of whom are very close to their sister. Also, Owen, who had always worked on or near the ocean, loves the sea and the city, and he is truly close to Louise's family. They have never had children.

While he has a deep sense of affection for his mother, he has never been terribly close to her, just as he hadn't been too close to his father. Owen had always respected his parents , but because he left home when he was 18 years old and has lived away from Moncton since then, he simply never felt feel a pressing need to be physically close. In addition, neither parent had ever taken to Louise, and they never could accept that he'd married a "damaged woman," as his father had referred to her.

When Dorothy had her fall, the seniors' home called Owen to tell him what had happened and that his mother appeared to be all right, even though she had been admitted to hospital. Owen immediately travelled to Moncton to see his mother and spent three days there —one of the days she was still in the hospital, and the other two back in her apartment.

Owen had seen his mother only once since his father's funeral, and he was surprised at how much she'd changed in three years. For one thing, Owen noticed how poorly his mother now moved; seldom would she even try to go from room to room without using at least a cane, and more often than not her walker. He attributed this to her recent fall and painful back. Then he noticed that she often confused dates, times, and events. This alarmed him because he remembered that she had taken care of all her own banking since his father died, though there was never that much to do. When he asked his mother about her financial situation and if anyone was helping her with it, Dorothy told him that whenever she needs money, she calls someone at the bank who transfers the amount to her friend Wilma's account at the same bank, and then Wilma withdraws it and gives it to her. She also said that she writes only a few cheques and that her rent to the seniors' home was deducted automatically. Other than that, there wasn't much banking to be done.

During Owen's visit, he and his mother had dinner together in the main-floor dining room. Although Dorothy had some difficulty walking even with her walker as a result of the spinal compression fracture, she wanted to be where most of the residents took their meals. During dinner Owen listened to his mother talk about some of the people she knew there. Even though she seemed to know something about most of them, she seemed to be vague about details. She also expressed veiled hints that perhaps some of the residents might be doing something wrong or, worse, illegal.

Owen spent most of his visit trying to arrange things for Dorothy so that she could maintain herself in the best possible way as she recovered from her injury. He requested some extra help in the room, including some bathing and dressing assistance. Dorothy initially declined this extra service, stating that she didn't need any help and that she didn't want anyone in her room for fear of having things stolen.

Over the course of his visit, Owen noted that he would have to repeat things he had told his mother over and over again because she kept forgetting what he'd said. But her memory for the "old days" was just fine, so he assumed that things could not be so bad if she could remember events from long ago and in such detail. When he went home, other than the concern about his mother's memory problems, he was feeling that all things considered, his mother was living safely and in relative comfort.

After his visit, Owen made sure he telephoned his mother once every two weeks for at least a few minutes. His conversations with her were relatively short, which didn't leave Dorothy much room to articulate in any detail any of her concerns or conditions. Owen didn't think he noticed any particular change in his mother, but he did sense that she acted as if he hadn't phoned before, and that she asked some of the same questions about himself and his life each time he called.

A few months after her accident, his mother did the totally unexpected—she called Owen. It was three in the morning and she wanted to know when his father was coming home because she knew for a fact that he and Owen were at some party without her. Her voice was very tense, and when Owen said none of what she claimed was true, reminding her that Jack had been dead for years, Dorothy yelled at him to shut up and stop lying to her.

A few months after her accident, his mother did the totally unexpected—she called Owen. It was three in the morning and she wanted to know when his father was coming home because she knew for a fact that he and Owen were at some party without her. Her voice was very tense, and when Owen said none of what she claimed was true, reminding her that Jack had been dead for years, Dorothy yelled at him to shut up and stop lying to her. Then she wanted to know how "his crazy wife" was, and Owen yelled back at his mother to stop talking like that and to listen. But she didn't. She just wanted to know over and over again when Jack would be back, and why Owen wouldn't help out and protect his aging, needy mother instead of going off to parties and living with some crazy woman.

By the time he got off the phone, Owen was devastated. First thing in the morning he called the head of the seniors' home and talked to the administrator. What he heard floored Owen. The administrator said that ever since her fall Dorothy had been on a gradual slide in her state of health. She explained to Owen that there were a number of problems and that the doctor was concerned that his mother had signs of dementia, most likely Alzheimer's disease. She reported that Dorothy was still able to get to the dining room by herself and do her own grooming, although sometimes the mix and match of clothes was a bit out of character for her — but no one seems to mind. And she was getting to the toilet on time, most of the time. But the administrator also told Owen that the staff was having someone help Dorothy with bathing all the time now, since she feels unsteady in the shower even though it has a chair in it to sit on.

The administrator suggested to Owen that he may want to try to visit more often and spend some time with his mother. She also reassured Owen that the seniors' home was equipped to care for people in Dorothy's situation, and that his mother was being moved to a floor where the staff could help residents with bathing, dressing, and, if necessary, preparing their food and sometimes even with feeding.

Owen then called the physician at the seniors' home. The doctor discussed some possible issues that might come up with Dorothy and suggested Owen talk about them with his mother "before it was too late."

Owen had never really discussed deep issues with his mother, having left home as a young adult. He wishes, now that his mother is failing and that he is not able to communicate with her in a more profound and and personal manner, that he'd done more to develop his relationship with her over the years. However, he does know that his mother is not a religious person and stopped attending church many years ago, saying to him that there was not much in it for her. She had always seemed a kind of "practical" person with no deep-seated sense of mystery or symbolism.

To Owen's surprise, when he did speak to his mother again, Dorothy was able to state quite emphatically that she would never want to be left a "vegetable," should she get seriously ill. She seemed able to clearly articulate her wish that if her condition couldn't be treated easily and the prognosis was that she couldn't return to her present state of physical or mental health, Owen should "let her go from this world." Owen was quite relieved to hear Dorothy state things so clearly. The doctor was able to reassure Owen that should Dorothy fall ill, Dorothy's wishes for minimal intervention of high-technology medicine would be respected. Owen told the doctor that he could be contacted in an emergency but that he trusted the physician's understanding of Dorothy's wishes if she were not able to express them at the time of a real medical crisis.

After these long-distance conversations, sitting in his small family room at the back of his frame house, Owen didn't know what else to do. He had to face his own personal challenges, and suddenly he had an added responsibility to manage. He knew that Dorothy was safe for the time being, and now he remains hopeful that he can provide sufficient support without having to leave home too often, because that is a physical, mental, and financial strain for him.

The Health Care Professional's Point of View

The first thing Owen must do is figure out what has happened to Dorothy. It appears that she is suffering from some form of dementia, such as Alzheimer's disease, and perhaps something else in addition to that disorder. It is also likely that she has been suffering from that condition for as long as a year prior to her fall. It does not seem likely that the fall itself caused her decline in mental function, but it is not uncommon for an acute medical event to lead to the recognition of dementia which a person may appear to have managed in his or her own environment for quite a while.

People with a moderate degree of dementia often succeed in managing their daily activities if they live in a reasonably supportive environment, such as a retirement home or seniors' building like the one in which Dorothy has been living. In Dorothy's case, for example, the staff at the bank have been very helpful to Dorothy, making sure that all financial transactions were conducted appropriately.

With a trauma like a fall, even if there is no head injury, which could potentially lead to a more rapid decline in mental function, the resultant hospitalization and need for analgesics containing codeine can increase the risk of a state of acute confusion, often referred to as delirium. This appears to be what happened to Dorothy. Although she made a reasonable recovery, the fact that the staff at the seniors' home has recommended an increased level of her personal care is an indication that her mental abilities are deteriorating.

If Owen were able to arrange it, Dorothy might benefit from a referral to a specialist in geriatrics, geriatric psychiatry or neurology. Whoever it is, it must be someone who has a lot of experience with older adults, especially those who have complex medical conditions and problems related to dementia of one sort or another. One goal would be to try and differentiate the possible causes of her dementia in order to take the best available steps to deal with the condition and the possible consequences of it. Also, the specialist physician can act as one of the resource people Owen should be able to turn to should his mother experience further decline.

By reviewing the events leading to the present state of affairs (the "history"), considering the physical findings, and running some tests (possibly a CAT scan or other brain imaging techniques and some blood tests), a physician may be better able to define the kind of dementia which has affected Dorothy. This process is important because age alone is not considered a basis for a decline in mental function in a manner that is affecting Dorothy. Although the likelihood of dementia increases substantially as one ages, it is still important to try and define all the possible confounding causes of the particular condition.

> *Although the likelihood of dementia increases substantially as one ages, it is still important to try and define all the possible confounding causes of the particular condition.*

For example, it is possible that the fall Dorothy experienced was due to a small stroke, not one large enough to cause paralysis but one that caused her to fall and accentuated the apparently rapid mental decline. It may be that she has blood pressure problems that were not noted previously or problems with her cholesterol. When all the findings are put together, the physician might be in a position to recommend treatments that could be useful in dealing with underlying risk factors that could cause further unwanted events.

If the physician believes that Dorothy is suffering from Alzheimer's disease, it may be worthwhile trying one of the new medications available for this condition. Although they have been in use for only a few years, the evidence suggests that for a reasonable percentage of patients with Alzheimer's-type dementia (and those with some variants of that condition), these drugs can improve the level of mental awareness and interactions with people. In addition, it appears that the drugs decrease the rate of further decline of the condition, thereby keeping patients in a more stable condition for a longer period of time.

Dorothy may respond to the medication, which could improve the way she functions and which would be a nice outcome of the drug intervention. But she may not respond and decline may continue despite any medical treatments. Dorothy could potentially become more agitated and the paranoia that Owen witnessed during that disturbing telephone call may become more apparent and interfere with her ability to function well in the social environment of the home in which she is presently living.

The next question Owen has to face is, where will his mother live as her condition deteriorates? The seniors' home claims it can provide a level of care called "assisted living," but should Dorothy need greater care than the facility and staff can provide, she would have to move to a nursing home. It would be worthwhile for Owen to visit some of the nursing homes in the vicinity and speak to the staff at Dorothy's home to find out what their experiences have been with the homes in the region. He should understand the process so he knows when to register her for admission, assuming there is a waiting list for some of the homes that he and Dorothy like. Owen needs to set his mother up in a reasonably safe and secure environment that will be able to handle the likely decline in her condition, especially since he lives so far away.

To make the best choice, Owen should discuss with the administrator of the home, as well as her family physician, all aspects of Dorothy's physical needs and stress that he wants his mother's stated wishes to be respected as she declines.

Visiting his mother is difficult for Owen, but he could arrange to speak to the nurse at the seniors' home once a week, just to catch up on things. He should also continue to call his mother, of course, and could establish a routine of always phoning on the same day at the same time so that his mother is more likely to remember. It would help put Owen's mind at ease if he could also arrange for a friend or neighbour in the seniors' residence to keep an eye out for Dorothy and to call Owen if there were ever any worries.

Like so many children who live far away from ailing parents, Owen has to cope as well as he can. All he can do – all anyone can do – is to try and do the best job possible.

CHAPTER ELEVEN

We're On Our Own:
How to Plan for the Future

A COUPLE IN THEIR MID-SIXTIES MUST consider how long and effectively they can care for an aging mother while planning the day they will retire and eventually require care themselves.

The Challenge

Jean and Frank Scott have lived on the outskirts of Peterborough, Ontario for more than 30 years, after having moved from Kingston where they were both born, raised, and educated. Jean is 62 and Frank is 65. Jean is a schoolteacher and plans to work until she retires at 65 because she loves her job and the kids, and she also wants to maximize her retirement pension. Frank runs the local hardware store. It has been a touch-and-go affair over the years, but it does have some value and Frank hopes to keep the store going and then, when the time is right, sell it and make some profit from the capital that's been invested in it. Jean and Frank also have some RRSPs and various modest investments that they have been putting away for their retirement.

They have many friends and neighbours in the surrounding area, but no children of their own. Jean has a sister who lives in Newfoundland with her family, and Frank has a brother and sister who still live in Kingston with their families. Jean's mother, Louise, aged 87, has lived with Jean and Frank since she lost her husband eight years ago. Her income is limited to little more than her OAS (Old Age Security) and GIS (Guaranteed Income Supplement).

Louise managed well until about a year ago when she fell and broke her hip and had some complications, including a stroke that was either caused by the fall or happened just after it. She was found to have an irregular heart beat and has since required coumadin (a blood thinner). She is also a longstanding diabetic, and for the past few years has required insulin injections.

Although Louise has made a good recovery from the fracture and the stroke, she's never really been the same since and can't help much around the house. In fact, she now needs help with several normal personal activities. Because Jean and Frank both work, and there is no other family nearby, they've been dependent on the Ontario home care system to help provide in-home support for Louise, including bathing and meal assistance and helping her with insulin injections and monitoring her blood sugar. Because Jean can get home from school by about 4 p.m. on the days she doesn't have after-school meetings, and Frank has some flexibility with the store when he has adequate help, they've managed with these limited care services provided through the local Community Care Access Centre (CCAC).

> *It will be a real challenge to make sure that Louise gets the services she needs without putting enormous pressure on Jean and Frank. They worry that they won't be able to afford to keep Louise at home should she deteriorate to the point that she requires full-time help.*

Early last fall, Frank and Jean received notice that the hours allotted to Louise's care were to be cut substantially because of funding restrictions to the CCAC by the provincial government. As a result, they've had to make some private arrangements with neighbours, friends, and number of local teenagers to fill in the gaps left by the reductions. They are paying for the assistance, but their real concern is not the financial drain; it is the prospect of what will happen should Louise require more care. It will be a real challenge to make sure that she gets the services she needs without putting enormous pressure on Jean and Frank. They worry that they won't be able to afford to keep Louise at home should she deteriorate to the point that she requires full-time help. Moreover, they've been thinking about what will happen to them during the next number of years, should they fall ill themselves and need social services

Since they don't have any children or other family in the vicinity, they've expressed these concerns to their physician and the social worker from the CCAC who worked with them in providing care for Louise. They're feeling very vulnerable in terms of their ability to cope with the needs of Louise physically and financially and at risk in terms of their own future.

The Health Care Professional's Point of View

There are two main issues involved here, the first being the very real and immediate anxiety about how to provide Louise with the best care possible while not putting Frank and Jean at emotional and financial risk. It is necessary for them both to continue working to maintain their income for as long as possible as their retirement pensions and savings are not sufficient to assure them a reasonably comfortable retirement for themselves, much less to assure that Louise's needs will be met in the future.

They should have a very frank discussion with Louise about the issues and options and let her know that they will do whatever they can to continue to look after her. But they must also tell her that if circumstances change and they cannot continue with this plan, they will look for a nursing home that is close by and suitable for her. They should make it clear that this plan is not meant to "abandon" Louise, but to make sure that they can continue to participate in looking after her and still preserve their energy.

> *Jean and Frank should make it clear that their plan is not meant to "abandon" Louise, but to make sure that they can continue to participate in looking after her and still preserve their energy.*

The financial implications may vary depending on Louise's income, but if she does not have anything beyond her OAS and GIS, there should be no other funding expected from Frank and Jean for her nursing home care. They would clearly take all the necessary steps to make sure the facility is the one most suited for her, and it is obvious from their history and relationship that they would visit her frequently and take part in as many social activities as possible, including taking her home for weekends and holidays whenever they could.

The second issue, Jean and Frank's concern about their own future, is more difficult to address. The future is always impossible to predict. Government policies could change so that society may become more senior-friendly. Access to necessary health care and social services may not be a major problem. Or, of course the opposite could become the case and those without supportive families or friends may be in deep trouble should things go wrong in terms of health or independence. What Jean and Frank can do, at least, is discuss their concerns with the family that they do have — their siblings and nieces or nephews — so that should they fall ill and need some support, their preferences are known.

Preparing a "living will," with the assistance of their physician, may help them feel comfortable with some of the difficult decisions that might be necessary in the future. Just naming a relative or close friend to be a surrogate decision-maker and making clear their hopes and expectations for a time when they can't make decisions for themselves could lesson the worries. If they are not sure they can count on anyone, they can turn to their lawyer and ask him or her to take on the role.

Some people move into retirement homes or seniors' residences to assure themselves some security and safety in their later years. In these communities, there is usually a way to get someone to agree to act as a support person or surrogate should the situation require it. So, although it is understandable to feel some anxiety, especially as they face the decline of Louise and the extra demands made on them, Frank and Jean can take many steps to assure themselves of safe and secure later years.

If the time comes when they are no longer able to look after Louise, Frank and June have to examine the options for long-term care for Louise, and there are many considerations. When looking for a long-term care facility, the options are often limited by geography. In some smaller communities there may be only one facility close by, and depending on the jurisdiction that facility may range from a retirement home with or without an assisted-living level of care to a regulated long-term care facility. Retirement homes usually fall under the category of unregulated homes because in most jurisdictions governments do not provide a regulatory framework under which such facilities function.

Some of the better homes of this nature belong to voluntary organizations that try and assure some reasonable level of quality of care — but staffing levels and services are not mandated by government. The facilities are usually privately run, sometimes as part of provincial or national chains. In some the quality of care is very high and the services personalized, but the cost, too, may be very high and there is usually no subsidy offered by government. Many retirement homes, especially those with assisted-living levels of care, provide services that in other situations are usually carried out by long-term care facilities, often known as nursing homes or homes for the aged.

In some jurisdictions there is a range of options within a framework of special care housing structures that also provide important and supportive care. There are various kinds of group homes for those with physical and/or psycho-social problems. Many facilities of this sort provide excellent care for individuals with special kinds of problems such as dementia of the Alzheimer's type.

When the option exists, many families try and get their loved one admitted to a regulated long-term care facility because the provincial government covers some of the costs and regulates the standard of care. The facilities themselves may be under the control of private for-profit corporations, government (usually municipal), or not-for-profit organizations. The last category often includes community organizations, religious, cultural or ethnic organizations, or those related to some common heritage or historical link. (These facilities are sometimes referred to as "charitable homes for the aged.") Many large cities have long-term care facilities that reflect the ethnic and cultural bias of that community. For example, in Toronto there are Catholic, Muslim, and Jewish homes for the aged as well as those that cater to the Chinese, Italian, Greek, Finnish, and Polish communities — to name just a few.

The attraction of the not-for profit facilities is the assumption that there is a source of commitment to the care of the elderly beyond that of financial profit. The standards of care and dedication may be better than those run by private companies that may be accountable to shareholders and other corporate interests. Having said that, there are certainly many for-profit organizations, some of which belong to large chains, that provide excellent service and quality care.

Probably the two most important considerations when choosing a long-term care facility are location and quality of care. Ideally the facility should be convenient to family members to enable them to visit easily and so that frequent short visits can take place, which are preferable to infrequent but longer visits.

Of course, the quality of care is paramount but can be difficult to assess. One worthwhile exercise is to ask other people who have loved ones living in the facility what they think. You can also ask if there has been an accreditation process and whether the facility has received accreditation or if you can access recent inspection reports. Of course, a visit to the facility to watch how residents are treated and the sense of pride that the staff demonstrates in what they are doing can give a pretty good idea about the standards of care and caring. However, sometimes quality of care can only be assessed after the fact, so close observation during the acclimatization process is crucial. How is your loved one progressing? How often does the staff meet with families? How accessible are they? Answering these questions may indicate the quality of care that is being provided.

When you move a loved one into a long-term care facility, it is worth finding out "who is who" in the staff hierarchy and who should be contacted for information and progress. Providing the staff with health care expectations is very useful. For example, if a living will exists, the staff should be provided with a copy, or at least be told of the person's wishes for treatment and care. A meeting with the assigned or chosen physician (depending on the situation) is always useful to make sure that both you and the doctor understand the general goals of care and the parameters around which medical care will be provided.

Some individuals are too frail and sick to be cared for in long-term care facilities. For example, individuals who require tube feeding or respirator care or complete bowel and bladder care or who are bedridden or semi-conscious may need to be in a chronic-care hospital, which has a different framework of care than what is provided in long-term care facilities. It is usually a medically based decision that results in admission to such a hospital-type facility. This may be as the first choice for admission or as a transfer from a long-term care facility should the person's condition deteriorate to the point that care can no longer be safely provided in the long-term care facility.

Choosing the right facility is very difficult for a family, and sometimes the bureaucratic process can be daunting to even the most informed. In some jurisdictions the decision-making process often appears very rushed to families struggling emotionally with the decisions. If possible, family members should seek the advice and assistance of a social worker who is knowledgeable in the field and familiar with the peculiar needs and preferences of the family. But, the difficult decisions have to be made, and whatever that decision is, the challenge is to make the best of it by being a loving and supportive family member and exploring ways to assist the staff and the facility fulfil their goal, to the best of their ability.

You may have the chance to join a family council or advisory group or volunteer to participate in recreational programs to augment the care and programs provided by the staff. Positive and engaged participation is usually far more productive and results in a better sense of dedication from the staff than constant complaining and finding fault, which unfortunately is the way that some families approach long-term care facilities. Constructive criticism is usually well received by a reputable organization, but more effective than criticism is a positive and participatory role of loving family members who help those directly in the caregiving role. Caring is infectious and staff usually recognize family members who do truly care for their loved ones, and they usually respond in a positive fashion which helps everyone.

Chapter Twelve

Finding a New Life:
Corrections and Concerns

MANY ELDERLY PEOPLE WHO HAVE LOST a spouse want to move forward and "get a life" at some point, yet often their children don't understand or approve. This inevitably leads to confusion and potential conflict.

The Challenge

When Don Benson died after a lingering illness, his wife, Nora, understandably grieved for more than a year and a half. They'd been married for 51 years, and it was a happy marriage throughout. They'd been extremely close—not just as husband and wife and parents, but as the closest of friends and confidants. In fact, while they'd had many friends and a very active social life, they always told everyone that the best free time was when they were alone together.

Nora found much comfort and solace in the support she got from her son, Jeremy, and daughter, Lisa, at the time of Don's death. They stayed very close to her for the first few months and, even after, kept a close watch over her. They visited and phoned frequently and brought her to their homes.

Some six months after the funeral, Nora told her children that she appreciated their kindness, but now she felt more stable and wanted some time to herself—to think about her life with Don, to sort things in the house, and to reflect. While Jeremy and Lisa at first worried that their mother was sliding into some kind of depression, they discovered, much to their relief, that she seemed to be all right being more on her own.

At the time of Don's death, Nora was still a relatively young "senior citizen" of 72 years. She was in good health; the only significant medical condition she'd had was cataract surgery three years earlier.

Jeremy at the time was 44 years old and working long hours as a fairly successful stock broker. Jeremy was married to Espeth, a very happy woman who worked part time at an upscale clothing boutique and who spent as much time as possible with their 11-year-old daughter, Dawn.

Lisa had just turned 40 when her father died. She lived in a common-law relationship with Marvin. They had no children, and they always explained that they'd never intended to have a family because both were devoted to their careers and each other. Lisa was an actress who regularly landed supporting roles in local playhouse productions and appeared in television commercials and print ads. Marvin was a graphic artist by day and an aspiring painter by night, working on canvases that were displayed in some of the smaller galleries and in various restaurants.

Both families got along well, despite being very different. And both really wanted to help Nora in any way they could.

During the time Nora wanted to spend more time alone, her children and their families pulled back, respecting her wish. Of course, they still visited her and invited her to visit them and spend time together during holidays and birthdays and other special events. Jeremy and Lisa each also spoke on the phone a couple of times a week with their mother.

As time passed, Nora seemed to regain her sense of confidence in herself and life in general. She spoke less of the "good times with Don" and more about how she was going to move into a retirement home in the next year or so, about the canasta card club she'd joined, about her church activities, or about a local book club that she was thinking of joining. In addition, she announced plans to become a volunteer at the local museum, a place that she always enjoyed.

Her children were amazed and thrilled at what they perceived as being a very healthy approach by their mother to the rest of her life. They also were delighted that Nora looked good; she dressed well, moved with comfort, and spoke clearly and lucidly about her life and day-to-day activities.

Six months ago, Nora told her children that she'd selected a retirement home and planned to sell the family home and move out within the year. She also surprised them with the news that she was going to take a seniors' bus tour across Canada that would last three weeks. She'd already signed up for the tour, which was departing a week after her announcement. Jeremy and Lisa asked their mother if she thought that was wise. Nora assured them it was perfectly safe, and told them with some sense of pride that she'd had her annual medical checkup recently and had been given a clean bill of health. And Nora reminded them how much she and Don used to enjoy going on bus tours and train rides and cruises.

And so Nora headed off, promising to not just send post cards, but to call either Jeremy or Lisa every few days. She did just that, and she always sounded cheerful and contented. The three weeks seemed a long time to her children, who worried about her since she'd never been on any trip alone before.

But Nora returned unscathed and unharmed. If anything, at the "welcome back" dinner they arranged for her she seemed brighter and happier than they'd seen her in a long time. It was during the dinner that Nora told her children and their spouses that her life had changed. She explained that a few months earlier she'd met a very nice widower at the canasta club, named Albert. He was 76 years old, tall, very considerate, and fun to be with. They'd had dinner together a few times. He was the one who suggested she go on the tour for which he had already signed up, and they'd just spent a lot of time together and were very comfortable with each other. He, too, liked reading and had joined the book club and thought that the museum volunteer activity was great fun. And he lived at the retirement home where she planned to move.

> It was during the dinner that Nora told her children and their spouses that her life had changed. She explained that a few months earlier she'd met a very nice widower at the canasta club, named Albert.

Jeremy and Lisa were flabbergasted, as were Espeth and Marvin. They had not expected this at all. They didn't know what to say as they exchanged glances across the dinner table. It was only when Nora asked what they thought that they each said it was a surprise.

Jeremy immediately wanted to know more about Albert —about his health, about his financial situation, about his family. He had a lot of questions that just bubbled out of him. Lisa remained very quiet and listened to her mother patiently talk about her new friend.

After Jeremy had taken Nora home, he called Lisa. They talked for quite a while, and agreed that this wasn't like their mother. They just couldn't imagine her finding someone else at this stage in her life. It simply didn't feel right to them, especially since their mother and father had been so close. Jeremy pointed out that he'd heard a lot of stories about widows and widowers who had "hit on" other elderly people in order to ensure their own comfort and financial security. He told her stories of stocks being transferred to such people in good faith, only to be cashed in and the person vanishing. It was an unsettling phone conversation for them both.

Lisa had yet another nagging concern, and she called her mother the next day to raise it. Lisa asked her mother how she really felt about this man; Lisa wasn't comfortable calling him by his name. Her mother responded that she felt very comfortable, and wanted to know why her daughter was asking. Lisa finally said that what was bothering her was that she loved her father and her memories of him, and her father and mother together, and she just couldn't see how Nora could toss all that aside and select another man.

Nora was stunned and hurt. She told her daughter that one had nothing to do with the other. She said that tears still came to her eyes and she felt an ache in her heart when she thought about Don, but there's nothing she could do to bring him back; she could only cling to the good memories. But, she reminded Lisa, she still had a life and she wanted to live it. Besides, she told Lisa, she and Albert were just friends, nothing more.

That didn't satisfy Lisa, and they ended the conversation on a tense note. Later, Lisa called Jeremy and reported what their mother had told her. Neither felt good about the developments, but nor did they know what to do about it. The only decision they made was that together the must convince their mother to abandon her friendship with Albert.

A few days later when Jeremy and Lisa went to see their mother to talk about their concerns, Nora became agitated and defensive and asked her children to let her have a life she could enjoy. They ended the session in a standoff—Nora determined to carry on with her plans, and Jeremy and Lisa equally determined to change her mind.

The Health Care Professional's Point of View

The death of a spouse often leads children to assume that the surviving parent will remain single and that their role as children will be to care and nurture the parent as a single widow or widower.

In many cultures the idea of remarriage is quite alien and many widows especially bear the mark of their status quite openly. It is unusual for them to reconnect for many reasons, including societal standards and family expectations. But in other cultures it is considered terrible for someone to be alone after the death of a spouse, and a lot of effort goes into trying to reconnect the person (especially in the case of widowers; the gender bias is clear).

In Canada and the rest of North America it is not uncommon for widows and widowers to remarry, although the likelihood for men is much greater than for women simply because there are many more older women then men. As well, our cultural bias finds it more acceptable for men to connect with much younger women than for women to take up with younger men.

So what's the problem with Nora's family? One would have thought that they would be delighted that their mother is in a position to have a meaningful relationship at this time of her life. But it is not uncommon for children to react exactly as Jeremy and Lisa have done. It would be useful for Jeremy and Lisa to explore the cause of their reaction so that they can come to understand it and prevent undermining their relationship with Nora or alienate her and her newfound "friend" who may some day become a more "significant other."

Children often have emotional reactions to situations that are based on assumptions or beliefs without looking at the situation from the perspective of the most important person affected by the situation, which in this case is Nora. Jeremy and Lisa seem to be forgetting that it is Nora's needs and wishes that should be paramount, and as much as possible they should be supporting her to be a physically and emotionally independent person. If they really thought about it, they would probably come to the conclusion that if either of them were struck by the tragedy of losing a spouse, they too might one day want to reconnect. Emotional and physical relationships are so central to human happiness and fulfillment that to deny such opportunities condemns people to a life of loneliness.

> *Jeremy and Lisa seem to be forgetting that it is Nora's needs and wishes that should be paramount, and as much as possible they should be supporting her to be a physically and emotionally independent person.*

A lot of children think of a parent's desire to reconnect as somehow compromising the respect and love for the deceased spouse. Yet if you ask those in loving relationships what they would want for their spouse if they died, most would say that the most important thing would be that their loved one not be left alone and that they should try and reconnect with someone else to share an emotional and physical relationship.

Some children are repelled by the thought that their parent might actually want to have sexual relations with another person, especially when they are older and after so many years with their other parent. Many younger people erroneously assume that human sexuality stops at a certain age. In fact the main barrier to healthy and fulfilling sexual relationships in the older years is the lack of a partner rather than the lack of desire or physical ability.

Lastly, there may be ulterior motives that the children are not expressing which are financial in nature. Sometimes a surviving parent is left with a lot of money and assets which the children assume will pass to them after the death of the surviving spouse. Therefore, a potential new spouse can be seen as a financial threat to an inheritance. It is also true that sometimes dishonest individuals prey on unsuspecting widows and widowers to take advantage of their financial situation, using their emotional relationship as the basis for poor financial decision-making. I have seen very few of these cases in my practice of more than 25 years, but indeed this might be a valid concern of children who want to be sure not only of their future inheritance but of the financial security of the surviving parent.

So what should the children do? Presumably they want to continue to have a loving relationship with their mother and at the same time assure their mother's happiness and their collective financial security. If they keep acting the way they are, they are not going to achieve their goals.

The first step is for them to sit down with Nora and express to her their support and happiness that she is finding her own life again and that they respect and love her for it. They should also say that they understand why it is so important that she find a potential partner for an emotional and, possibly a physical relationship. They must emphasize their support for her happiness as a major priority in their lives.

With that said, they can then say that they just want to be sure that whatever is done does not put Nora at any risk, emotionally, physically, or financially. They should offer to meet Albert and arrange a time where they can do so in a relaxed manner and welcome him as a special visitor and person in their mother's life The more they include him in family events, the more likely they will be able to figure out what kind of person he is and how he and Nora seem together.

With that kind of approach Jeremy and Lisa will be in a much better position to express other opinions and concerns. For example, they might suggest that should the relationship develop into something more serious or legally binding, Nora should seek the advice of a lawyer to make sure that her financial resources are protected. In addition, if Nora wants to protect her children's financial inheritance as well, there are legal ways of doing so. Taking such a step would probably go a long way in soothing the suspicions and concerns that the children might rightfully have, but may not be able to articulate to themselves or to Nora as they contend with this new situation.

Many older people reconnect very successfully in their later years, especially after the loss of a long-time spouse. What more wonderful thing could happen to a person who would otherwise spend their remaining years dependent on their children and friends? A new partner does not desecrate the honour of the previous spouse; if anything, many people who have been through such experiences find that they can share the importance of the previous relationship and use it as a basis for a new and fulfilling relationship. Children can play an important role in supporting and encouraging their parents' independence and need for emotional and physical fulfillment, an essential part of human existence.

CHAPTER THIRTEEN

Decision Time:
Planning for the Inevitable

WHEN ONE PARENT IS ILL AND the other parent appears to be unable to make appropriate caregiving choices, the children must make some hard decisions about what steps to take to protect the dignity and well-being of both.

The Challenge

Margit and Tamas Ujhazy were childhood sweethearts. They were born in the same small village in Hungary, and they married when she was 16 and he was 19. A few years later, they emigrated to Saskatchewan when Canada was encouraging people to come to work in this country. Under the terms of the agreement with the government, for the first five years they had to work on a farm—which is what they did back in their native Hungary. After the five-year period expired, they moved to Esterhazy where they rented a room in a private home and worked in the area—he as a farmhand, and she as a domestic.

They never prospered, but lived frugally, and when Margit was expecting their first child they bought a tiny four-room bungalow that has been their home since the late 1950s.

Now, Margit is 70 and Tamas is 73. Margit had a serious stroke a year ago that has left her totally incapacitated and in need of round-the-clock care in a nursing home. She is able to speak, but not easily, and often mixes English with Hungarian. Meanwhile, Tamas continues to live in their home and work part time at a local hardware store.

They have two children—Elizabeth, now 40, and Arpad, 37. Elizabeth, a radiologist, lives in Vancouver with her second husband, Bob, a software programmer. Arpad, a chartered accountant with a consulting firm, lives in Edmonton with his wife, Nancy, and their three children. Since leaving home, neither Elizabeth nor Arpad has been very close to each other or to their parents, but since their mother's stroke, both siblings have taken a more active involvement with their parents and with each other.

When their mother suffered her stroke, Tamas called his children—something he'd not done in more than a decade—to tell them what had happened. Both Elizabeth and Arpad went to Esterhazy to see their mother and visit with their father. It was Elizabeth's first visit home in more than five years and Arpad's first time back home in four years. Elizabeth and Arpad now call their father every Sunday and stay in touch with each other through weekly e-mails to compare notes about what Tamas has told them.

Recently, their mother was diagnosed with bone cancer. Tamas told them about the diagnosis in one of their weekly telephone calls, but said that everything was under control. In a subsequent telephone conversation, he told Elizabeth that nursing home staff had complained that Margit yells a lot, and that they think that she's in extreme pain. But, Tamas said, she's not really in much pain at all; rather, all the noise she's making and the claims of pain are her way to get more attention.

Elizabeth asks her father who their family doctor is, and decides to call her. When they eventually connect, the doctor tells Elizabeth that Margit is indeed in extreme pain, which is why she's often yelling out. The doctor wants to place her on morphine patches, but explains that Tamas refuses to agree and, at most, allows only Tylenol #3 to be administered. The doctor also tells Elizabeth that Tamas, who's been diagnosed with early signs of Alzheimer's, proudly points out that his wife has a history of bearing pain very well. Tamas has said that while everything possible should be done to keep Margit alive, morphine patches are unacceptable. It's not clear to the doctor why that's the case.

Now Elizabeth and Arpad face a dilemma. The doctor has explained Tamas's wishes and suggested that their father may not be making choices in a sound frame of mind. Elizabeth and Arpad agree that Arpad should see their father and talk about what needs to be done for both their parents. Uncertain of what they should do about either parent, the two siblings decide that their father's views should be sought and, if they make sense, applied.

When Arpad meets his father in Esterhazy, he is told that his mother often took to yelling out loud when she felt she was in pain, but that this was a natural over-reaction that shouldn't be taken seriously. His father reminds Arpad how much and how loud his mother used to yell even if she just bumped an elbow into a door or got a slight cut on a finger. Arpad can't remember any yelling at all by his mother, so while he wants to believe his father, he's very conscious that his mother is suffering terribly from her bone cancer, while incapacitated by her stroke.

No matter how much he talks to his father during his weekend visit, Arpad can't convince him to approve the morphine patches or any other pain management assistance for his mother. And the more they talk, the more Arpad realizes his father is at times very logical and lucid, but at other times he is seemingly confused and uncertain of past events. Arpad wants to believe his father, yet he's torn by nagging doubts and a growing concern for his mother's condition. By the end of the weekend, Arpad feels the visit was an exercise in futility, and that even if his mother has a low pain threshold, that's got nothing to do with the fact that she's got bone cancer, which he recalls is one of the most painful types of cancer there is.

When Arpad returns home, he calls his sister and they have a long discussion about what they can and should do for both their mother and their father. Both realize that there is little they can do long-distance, and that neither really wants to take on the responsibility of becoming a dedicated family caregiver. They exchange stories of their childhood and teenage years that demonstrate their parents didn't do as much as they should have for either of them—and then they realize that they are groping for a justification to do little or nothing.

Ashamed, agitated, and confused, Elizabeth and Arpad finally decide that they must try to help make their mother's suffering as manageable

> *Ashamed, agitated, and confused, Elizabeth and Arpad finally decide that they must try to help make their mother's suffering as manageable as possible, and that they need to try to deal with their father and find a way to get him the help he'll need when their mother dies and as his Alzheimer's continues to develop and affect him.*

as possible, and that they need to try to deal with their father and find a way to get him the help he'll need when their mother dies and as his Alzheimer's continues to develop and affect him.

The Health Care Professional's Point of View

Elizabeth and Arpad face a situation in which there really isn't a "right" answer, but they have to struggle with weighing the implications of whatever difficult decision they make. Here they have one parent who appears to be suffering unnecessarily from pain due to cancer and another whose dignity they are trying to respect, even as he shows evidence of cognitive decline. The respect for one parent's needs appears to be in direct conflict with that of the other parent. As both children try to show respect for their parents, they must struggle with the impact of whichever decision they make.

To ignore the need for proper pain management in a parent suffering from malignant bone pain seems cruel and unacceptable to them. However, since their father is the person making decisions, they are trying to respect him even though the consequences for their mother are not acceptable emotionally, nor are they acceptable as part of a standard of medical practice for palliative care.

For most health care professionals, withholding pain control in the palliative stage of malignant disease is considered abrogating one's professional responsibility. Therefore, in order for the children to care for their mother and try to maintain respect for their father, they are going to require enormous sympathy and assistance from the health care professionals that are caring for both of their parents.

If, indeed, Tamas is showing evidence of cognitive impairment, this should be formally addressed by his physician. It might be that the diagnosis is incorrect and that there is another explanation for the change in his personality and judgment-making process. For example, depression can appear to cause memory lapses, when in fact the cognitive changes are an outcome of the depressive disease. Some medications can also cause lapses in cognition, memory, and judgment (such as sleeping pills and sedatives), and this possibility should be evaluated in an objective fashion, rather than be left for the children to surmise what might be going on.

If after appropriate review, assuming that Tamas agrees to the evaluation (which can be facilitated by the assistance of his physician if the situation is explained by the children), it is found that there is no clear clinical explanation for his views and no disorder is found that might compromise has ability to be a surrogate decision-maker, the children are really faced with a problem. They will have to get as much assistance as possible by physicians and nurses whom their father trusts to try and help him understand the importance of proper pain management for their mother. It would be worth exploring why he is opposed to morphine patches. If he is concerned about her becoming addicted or overly somnolent, perhaps alternatives to pain management might be suggested that he will not perceive as risky or that might "end Margit's life." This might include a less potent analgesic given on a round-the-clock basis coupled with drugs such as tricylclic antidepressants that can accentuate the effects of analgesics.

If their father still refuses some appropriate regimen of pain management, then the children will have to decide whether they should apply to replace their father as surrogate decision-maker because of his failure to fulfill this role according to most legal frameworks (i.e., acting in the best interests of the person on whose behalf you are acting). This will not be an easy decision and could potentially cause a rift, temporary or otherwise, in the relationship between Elizabeth and Arpad and their father.

If, on the other hand, it is found clinically that their father is cognitively impaired and incapable of making proper surrogate decisions, he can be replaced by the children. This may result in a negative response from him, the only difference being that the children can perhaps get some help from the physician in explaining why surrogacy has to be changed. In that way, the doctor can bear some of the responsibility for the decision, and then proper decisions concerning Margit's palliative needs can be met without the children appearing to be going against the wishes of their father.

> *The children must be prepared for the likelihood that after their mother dies, their father is going to require an extra measure of help.*

The children must be prepared for the likelihood that after their mother dies, their father is going to require an extra measure of help. If he is, indeed, in the process of manifesting evidence of dementia and early Alzheimer's, he may feel the loss of his wife profoundly and his symptoms may be exaggerated. It is likely that he will need help in his home. Or perhaps the need may arrive for him to live elsewhere. Such a decision should not be taken precipitously, but in a measured manner, as the mourning period may be prolonged.

The hope is that their father's dignity can be maintained as much as possible while they still meet the first imperative, assuring themselves that their mother has a peaceful and pain-free death.

CHAPTER FOURTEEN

End of Life:
Caring and Sharing

IT'S NATURAL FOR CHILDREN TO BECOME intensely concerned and involved when a parent is in the process of dying, let alone when the other parent isn't well. The real challenge is to know how to become constructively involved rather than intrusive.

The Challenge

Simon Delacroix is 73 years old and dying of lung cancer. His wife, Emma, is the same age. Because she's a severe diabetic and more than 40 pounds overweight, as well as being physically and mentally exhausted from trying to care for her husband the past two years, Emma is incapable of caring for Simon with the level of intensity required.

They live in Windsor, Ontario in their three-bedroom suburban home. They now have regular help with lawn and snow care. As Simon's condition continues to deteriorate and Emma is ever less capable of caring for him in their home, even with daily tasks, they've turned to the local Community Care Access Centre (CCAC) for additional support. With budgetary constraints, that support is nominal—a homemaker who comes to help bathe Simon and do some light housecleaning twice a week for two hours each visit.

Simon and Emma have one child, Allison, who is 46 years old. She lives in London, Ontario—a bit less than a two-hour drive away—with her husband, Daryl, and their two children, Melissa and Mary. Allison works as a bank teller, and Daryl is a program director with the city's parks and recreation department. Allison has tried to help her parents as best she can, but Simon and Emma have been stubborn all along, consistently rejecting her repeated pleas to have her father put in a nursing home so he can get the attention and services he needs and to reduce the pressure on her mother.

Simon, Emma, and Allison and her husband are fully cognizant that Simon will probably die within the next four to six months according to their family doctor and the oncologist who's been examining him. However, the family is having a very difficult—nearly impossible—time talking about it in any constructive fashion. They're frozen in inaction.

Simon is in a state of denial. He rationalizes his terminal condition and most days proclaims that "this is the first day of the rest of my life, and I'm going to improve." While this may seem a positive mental attitude, with Simon it's actually a deep longing to regain his health while wishing away the reality of the situation.

Emma, meanwhile, is angry that Simon didn't stop smoking years ago when she did. She blames him for being on the verge of a premature death, and while trying to make him as comfortable as possible, she too often verbally attacks him for his selfishness and lack of self-control. Emma is emotionally distraught, and she is also worried about her own health, placing the blame directly on her husband for the state of their lives.

And instead of appreciating Allison's concerns and expressions of support, both parents blame their daughter for meddling in what they believe is their own problem. They can't see her as the adult she is. Allison, in their minds, is still the child who should listen to their words and wisdom and show respect for their wishes, which are entrenched in a paradigm of parent-child control.

Allison is totally frustrated and angry with her parents. She's determined to help her father die with dignity and with the most support possible. Yet, whenever she calls (daily) or visits (weekly), her father argues that he's in stable condition and on the road to recovery. Meanwhile, Allison's mother continues to complain that her father is his own worst enemy, rejecting all the positive things she's doing to help him. Emma often tells Allison that her father actually deserves to suffer because he's so long ignored all the good advice that she, their doctor, and even their friends have given him.

From Allison's perspective, her father is just ignoring reality and not planning for his own death. Her mother is hurting as a result of her husband's inevitable impending death and her own anger. And no one is doing any planning that will reduce the amount of pain and uncertainty that's about to happen in their family.

Allison is totally frustrated and angry with her parents. She's determined to help her father die with dignity and with the most support possible. Yet, whenever she calls or visits, her father argues that he's in stable condition and on the road to recovery.

Allison doesn't have power of attorney for either parent, although she's talked about it with both of them a number of times the past few years. Nor does she have any other legally binding rights to make decisions on behalf of either parent. In short, legally, Allison has no say in what happens with either parent, and that probably won't change.

She's also spoken several times to her parents' family doctor. In his seventies, the doctor treats her the same way her own parents do —with a level of disdain and distance, talking down to her rather than with her. He always concludes conversations with assurances that everything is "under control" and that he knows what's best for her father and her mother. Meanwhile, in conversations with the case manager at the CCAC , Allison gets the distinct impression that she's talking to a stressed, overworked, well-intentioned but overwhelmed professional who is trying to provide the services she can while meeting her many other obligations within the constraints she must face every day.

The Health Care Professional's Point of View

The challenge to children of aging parents is to try and provide care and concern while respecting their parent's option to do it "their way." When you think about it, it is the same challenge parents face when their children are growing up: to allow them to make decisions and do things that may seem to fly in the face of their best interests and may not reflect the opinions and advice of their parents.

In some child-parent relationships, the conflict in values and opinions is so great that their relationship is disrupted for many years, if not for life. Usually, as children mature, they begin to understand and accept their parents better and usually, but not always, parents understand their children. Some parents can never get out of the mold of treating their children as children, rather than as adults who happen to be their offspring.

So what can Allison do? First she must accept that the most she can achieve is to give her best care and advice to her parents, and then let them make their own decisions, even if they are not the best ones possible. In terms of getting that message across to her parents, it is probably worthwhile trying to meet with them to tell them that, as part of her love and devotion to them, she wants to do whatever she can to help. She can say that her perspective on what is going on may be different from theirs, but that she is willing to accept their views. She should say that while she wants to help, she will not interfere with their decision-making but will be available if necessary when they need her.

Allison might suggest to her mother that blaming her father for what has happened does nothing to help the situation, but may in fact make things worse. However, if it is her mother's nature to look for blame, then Allison is not going to get very far with that approach, other than trying to focus her mother's efforts on what is necessary to make her father as comfortable as possible.

As for the physician, Allison is not likely going to get very far with her pursuits with him. But it may be worthwhile writing to him and thanking him for all the years of support that he has provided to her parents and family. She should express her concerns about her father's present and future needs, and at the same time acknowledge that the doctor may understand her father well and that she will trust that he will make the right decisions if and when they are necessary.

Allison also may want to ask the CCAC what kind of home care might be available should her father decide that he does not want to enter a palliative care unit—or for that matter, any other kind of facility—no matter how bad things are.

It is not uncommon for people suffering from cancer to deny their disease, and trying to convince them of the truth may be counter-productive. Most terminal cancers progress to a point where the person suffering is no longer able to deny the illness because of the symptoms. But, the element of hope should never be taken away from someone who realizes that he or she has a terrible disease. That may mean for the family that the focus is on relieving symptoms, rather than trying to cure the disease. Sometimes something urgent or acute happens that "shakes" the person suffering from the disease into reality. For example, with lung cancer it could be bleeding from the lung. Or it could be evidence that the cancer has spread to the bone, causing great pain, or to the brain, causing seizures or headaches. Whatever it is, the shift in symptoms that cannot be ignored may help everyone focus on the reality of the illness and on the future.

At this point, Allison has to find ways to avoid getting angry with her mother for being angry and frustrated herself. She can be supportive of her mother while not taking on the responsibility of trying to ensure a particular plan of approach. By removing the sense of responsibility for the outcome, Allison may be able to participate in the care of both her father and her mother without feeling that she has "failed" just because things do not go the way she would want them to go.

Unless there is a sudden turn for the worse, a time will likely come when Allison will be able to provide support and care for her parents. It may be necessary to take a more passive approach right now so that her parents can work out their issues as a couple, however abnormally she may think they are doing it. She should continue to visit on a regular basis, but not be judgmental when she does. She should call on a periodic basis and, again, listen a lot but not give advice unless it is asked for.

When her parents are ready for her help, she can then be there without resentment. It is crucial for her to not blame them for what has happened and for not allowing her to be involved when she thinks it is necessary. The timing, within reason, has to be their timing, and she has to accept that she can only do what she can do and, of course, what she wants to do, which is to provide the best love and support she can in this very difficult situation.

Meanwhile, Alison should prepare herself for her father's death.

One of the difficult experiences that children likely will face when a parent is nearing the end of life is dealing with the reality and the anticipation of loss, while trying to maintain the relationship with the still-living person. Some children and other family members and sometimes friends withdraw from the person as a way of dealing with the coming loss of a loved one. One often hears people who say, "I couldn't face the experience. I would have nothing to say and I was afraid of breaking down". Some individuals find ways to relate and communicate in the deepest and most profound and loving way to their family and friends when they are dying, while others project anger and sorrow and repel those who try to express their love.

For children and other family members, it is important to recognize that the knowledge of impending death is not easy, even for the most exceptionally balanced and emotionally secure individuals. It is important to overcome whatever hesitation may exist in visiting and being with the person as he or she nears the end. The issue is not about the feelings of the person doing the visiting, but about that of the person who is being visited. Most people do not want to be alone when they are dying, even though some act in a way that appears to push away even those they love. It is usually valuable to make a point of visiting, and if possible in a predictable fashion so that the person can count on the visit and have something to look forward to. It is not necessary to do anything elaborate when visiting but sometimes a nice small gift, especially of something the visitor knows the one they are visiting might value, is often very much appreciated.

> *For children and other family members, it is important to recognize that the knowledge of impending death is not easy, even for the most exceptionally balanced and emotionally secure individuals.*

The next question is, what does one do during the visit? The answer is, "just be there". That might include talking about anything, big or small but usually personal on a positive note—what is happening to friends and children that the visitor believes their loved one would enjoy hearing. Bringing pictures that reflect good experiences are also usually welcome with the intention of helping the person continue to participate in the positive aspects of life. When asked by family members if they should be emotional, I usually tell them if that is the way they feel, then it is okay, but to always remember it is the person who is ill who is the centre of the exercise, not them. I usually encourage families to let their loved one know just how wonderful a person they are and how meaningful they are and always will be to those who love them.

Lastly, I recommend to families to do as much touching as possible: holding a hand, giving a kiss, and providing a soothing massage if that seems to be welcome and helpful. Do not expect the person to necessarily respond in kind, which is not important. This is a time for giving on the part of family and friends and not expecting anything in return from the person who is ill and coming to terms with his or her own impending death. After it is over, those who were able to give of themselves and be patient with impatience and express affection and devotion will reap the benefits for many years after the event. They can usually find comfort in the way they behaved at the end, even when the loss is great and the loved one is no longer with them.

CHAPTER FIFTEEN

Moving On:
Living Life without a Loved One

IT'S NOT EASY LEARNING HOW TO cope with the grieving, how to live on when a spouse or a parent dies, and how to deal with the trauma, guilt, and pain that's involved.

The Challenge

Marilyn O'Connor is a recent widow. Her husband, Conrad, died six months ago. Although everyone knew that Conrad's death was inevitable and it was just a matter of how long he could hold out against the pancreatic cancer, his actual passing still came as a shock. Marilyn, her son, Wes, and stepdaughter, Wendy, and their families and several dozen friends attended a graveside service for Conrad on a dreary, overcast fall day with on-and-off again rain showers that matched their own feelings.

For two months before his death, Conrad had been a patient at a palliative care unit at their local hospital. Marilyn, 68 years old, spent hours with her 72-year-old husband every day. And while many nights she had a series of friends spend time visiting with her and offering support, Marilyn was deeply troubled and very afraid of life without Conrad.

For both, this was their second marriage. Marilyn had left her first husband some three decades ago, because of his alcohol problem and concerns about herself and her son's well-being. She managed to get herself back into the stream of things as a single mother and did well with her new job in an advertising agency.

Conrad's wife died when her car hit black ice on December 24, 1968. She was killed instantly in the crash, but their two-year-old daughter, Wendy, survived with just a few bruises and a long-lasting confusion about what happened to her mother.

Marilyn and Conrad met at a wedding in 1972: she attending as a friend of the bride, and he as a relative of the groom who was at the last moment pressed into serving as best man. It seems the groom and his intended best man had a major disagreement just days before the wedding, and so Conrad was recruited.

A few weeks after meeting at the wedding, Conrad called Marilyn to see if she and her young son would like to join Wendy and him at an Easter egg hunt. So the relationship began, growing into a warm, comfortable friendship, and then into a strong emotional attachment.

Two years after meeting—and over time finding that their children got along amazingly well—Conrad proposed. Three months later, they were married at a simple ceremony attended by a handful of friends.

In the years since the marriage, Marilyn and Conrad grew very close to each other and their children. During the summer months, the family often went camping together, and each winter Marilyn and Conrad would go on what they used to call a "just us" holiday for at least a week to a Caribbean island or some other warm vacation spot.

They were not rich, but they were comfortable. Conrad was a partner in a small law firm, and Marilyn continued working part time in the creative department of the same advertising agency where she had started after leaving her first husband. Meanwhile, Wes and Wendy emerged as good kids who grew into serious college students and responsible adults. Conrad often told his friends that he and Marilyn were extremely fortunate to have two such wonderful kids. Wes was married at age 30 to Amy, the daughter of Vietnamese refugees; they have two daughters and live in Edmonton. Wendy was married when she was 27 to Mark, who was just establishing his dentistry practice in Toronto, and four years later she gave birth to their only child, Damian.

Conrad retired precisely on his 65th birthday; Marilyn had stopped working 10 years earlier, instead spending time in volunteer work. Until he was diagnosed with his cancer, they travelled as much as possible, played golf together, spent a lot of time hiking in forests, and had a quiet but satisfying social life.

When they retired, Conrad and Marilyn decided to live in Orillia, an hour's drive north of Toronto, but within short driving distance of many golf courses and large parks for hiking. The retirement years were good to them, and for them. Conrad, always an animal lover, became involved in the local humane society as a volunteer and fundraiser, but because they wanted to be free to travel, they decided not to have an animal of their own.

The pancreatic cancer was a real blow to them all. It was totally unexpected, and right from the outset their family doctor and the oncologist who was seeing Conrad made it clear that the prognosis was very poor. In fact, the oncologist strongly recommended not operating and suggested that any form of treatment was not going to be beneficial in any way. For the first few months, they decided to not tell Wes or Wendy about the cancer, but then thought better of it and explained to them and their spouses, Amy and Mark, exactly what the situation was.

The family rallied in support of Conrad. Amy and Mark's own parents—with whom they'd always been on very good terms—would call often to see how Conrad was doing, and they stayed in touch with regular e-mails. Wendy, who lived in Toronto, visited her father every other day and helped her stepmother with housework, and Wes called him at least two or three times a week just for a few minutes.

However, it was clear that Conrad was in a rapid state of decline, with ever-increasing pain that was being treated with increasingly stronger doses of morphine and other pain relievers, given by mouth, injection, or patches. It was also clear that caring for him at home was becoming more and more difficult for Marilyn.

Watching Conrad in his pain and seeing him virtually shrink before their eyes was painful for Marilyn and Wendy. The oncologist finally suggested that they consider placing him in the palliative care unit. This was devastating for Marilyn to hear, but after talking it over with Wendy and Wes, she agreed it seemed like the best thing to do. Although the admission process was painful to them, the assistance of the unit's social worker, Cynthia, did make some of the decision-making easier.

Near the end, Marilyn was allowed to stay over in the special family room at the palliative care unit. Emotionally she was exhausted, and by the time Conrad died, she hardly had any tears left to shed. Cynthia was very supportive of Marilyn and a few times during the final days she gave Marilyn the opportunity to talk out her feelings about the loss she knew she was going to experience. Wendy resigned herself to the inevitable, but still wanted to find some element of hope to cling to.

Wes flew to Toronto the day his stepfather died, arriving at the palliative care unit just hours before the end. Neither Wendy nor Wes had much contact with Cynthia, although she did offer to meet with them if they wanted to. They declined.

After the funeral, Marilyn found there was a huge empty space in her life. She became withdrawn and very quiet. She rejected her friends' offers of company, choosing instead to spend hours looking at old photos and videos of her holidays with Conrad.

> *After the funeral, Marilyn found there was a huge empty space in her life. She became withdrawn and very quiet.*

Wendy spent weeks in a very depressed state, and kept questioning why her father's condition wasn't diagnosed sooner, and why more couldn't have been done for him. She called her stepmother every day, e-mailed back and forth with Wes, and found that she was having a difficult time concentrating on her work. Mark offered as much support as possible, but his practice kept him busy six days a week, so he was limited to doing the best he could consoling her and trying to spend more time with Damian.

Three months after the funeral Mark found his wife was still incapable of getting back to what he thought should be their normal life, and he saw that Marilyn was also still in a deep state of grieving. Mark suggested to Wendy that some counselling would be helpful. This caused a huge outburst of anger from Wendy, who lashed out at Mark for not understanding because his parents were still well and together, while her father was dead just when he was beginning to enjoy his life.

Wes, meanwhile, seemed more collected, but in their weekly telephone conversations, Mark felt that he, too, was still in pain, but just burying it.

The Health Care Professional's Point of View

Dealing with death is not easy. It doesn't matter what a person's background and experience might have been, the death of a loved one is a major challenge to a person's equilibrium. However, since death is intrinsic to life, everyone eventually has to come to terms with the realities of someone they love dying.

What can family and friends do to help with the process of bereavement and grief? This is not any easy question to answer, but there are people with a lot of experience in the field and there are processes that have been proven to be helpful to those going through the experience.

Many religions and different cultures have traditions that allow families to mark the various periods of time related to death so that social networks can be re-established with the view of reintegrating family members back into life. In other cultures, the role of the bereaved spouse is almost institutionalized so that there are barriers to reintegration back into the social fabric of the community.

> *Before anything can be done for Marilyn and her family, someone has to recognize that something is not right and probe possible avenues to improve the situation. The idea is not to try to forget the pain of death and loss, but rather to turn it into something positive that provides a reason once again to participate in life's activities.*

Before anything can be done for Marilyn and her family, someone has to recognize that something is not right and probe possible avenues to improve the situation. The idea is not to try to forget the pain of death and loss, but rather to turn it into something positive that provides a reason once again to participate in life's activities. Many palliative care units, because of their recognition of the difficult path that family members often take after the loss of a loved one, offer bereavement services and counselling to assist family members.

It would have been nice if the palliative care unit where Conrad was a patient had such a program. It may be that it does, but for some reason no contact has been made by the appropriate person to Marilyn or

Wendy, as the two of them seemingly are having the worse part of the grieving experience. If Wes is the person most likely to be able to take some initiative in helping Marilyn and Wendy accept assistance, it might be worth his speaking to a member of the palliative care unit's staff to explore what options exist.

Most palliative care programs have social workers involved in the care and support of family members. It is this person, especially if the family has had a good relationship with that person during the dying process, who can become a link in the process of working through the grieving period. Since there was a social worker involved in Conrad's hospitalization, and because Marilyn had the most contact with her, the logical place to start might be to approach Cynthia about the possibility of calling Marilyn. She could ask how things are going and invite Marilyn for a chat as part of the hospital's bereavement program. Wes could call Cynthia and explain what is going on and ask what might be done to help especially Marilyn and Wendy.

Cynthia's overtures might be rebuffed and thought to be intrusive. However, most social workers and counsellors who deal with bereavement are pretty good at managing an initial rejection of offers for assistance. On the other hand, most people experiencing grief understand that life has to go on and usually respond to gentle and caring overtures for help. Counselling can help normalize the psychological and physical symptoms often associated with grieving and create a safe environment to explore painful feelings. Even when death is expected and family members are prepared for the final event, the grief reaction may not be any less intense or prolonged than when a death is sudden.

Loving and caring family members can be instrumental in such assistance, although the kind of response that Mark experienced from Wendy is not that unusual. The timing of the next approach to begin discussion has to be carefully considered and prepared for and could be couched in the desire to help deal with the next stages of life. Mark has to be sensitive to Wendy's sensibilities, but he can build on being able to help her stepmother, while being available for each other and their child.

Each situation is different, but the goal has to be to regain meaning in life, which does not imply forgetting the person who has died and who was loved. Sometimes a way can be found to commemorate the person who died to give extra meaning to survivors. That is often why endowment funds for students, projects, or donations to charitable societies are suggested as a way of remembering the life of a loved one.

The wife of one of my patients decided to set up an endowment fund in her husband's name for the psychiatry unit that was so helpful in his overcoming severe depression. He spoke about it very highly after he recovered from his mental illness, prior to his death from another cause. In addition, she decided to become a volunteer at the hospital in which the psychiatry unit was located so that she could help other people.

In this case, Marilyn might want to consider setting up a fund for the palliative care unit to provide a better place for families to stay during the final days of their loved one's life. Or she might offer to work for the Cancer Society as a canvasser or in its office. This kind of work often allows for relationships to develop with other people who have lost loved ones to cancer; this common bond against the "enemy" of cancer often leads to social involvement.

Another option might be for Marilyn to get involved with the humane society as Conrad had, and continue with an activity that was dear to his heart. Similar options might be attractive to Wendy, although the main focus appears to be to meet the needs of Marilyn. It is possible that if her needs are met, Wendy will refocus her energies on the future rather than the past.

Whatever is done, the family has to be sensitive to the needs of Marilyn and Wendy, especially as they seem to be having the greatest difficulty. It is not that Wes might not benefit from bereavement counselling, it is just that he may have to get involved after the pattern and process is already established with his mother and sister.

The goal, of course, is to "get on with life" because that is what life is all about. Those people who do not accomplish that goal often become embittered and lose the ability to enjoy and share life. with others.

It seems that if Conrad knew what was happening he would tell his family to remember him as someone who enjoyed life and that what he would want is that they continue to live in a loving and expansive way. His death should be a catalyst to them to remember the wonderful things in life and to strive to enjoy them rather than be a reason to dwell on the past and the sadness that it contains.

Roz and Max
by
Michael Gordon

MY FATHER'S VOICE WAS SHAKY, "MOMMY had a little stroke and is in the hospital. They called it a 'transient' attack."

My 82-year-old father, Max, was calling me in Toronto from Brooklyn where he and my mother Roslyn (Roz), also 82, lived together in the cottage-like home they had owned for almost 40 years. He explained that my mother had suddenly had trouble speaking and her face had gone crooked. By the time she arrived at the hospital by ambulance she had recovered, but was admitted for testing.

As a geriatrician practising in Toronto I knew that my mother, a diabetic, had atrial fibrillation and was at risk for a so-called embolic stroke (blood clot to the brain). The cardiologist explained that her CAT scan was normal and that he had anticoagulated her (thinned the blood). He was trying to convince her to go on a long-acting anticoagulant, called Warfarin, but she was adamant that she didn't want that drug because of the risks of bleeding and the need for frequent blood tests. I was not surprised that my mother, a very active and spry person, would not want to be encumbered by frequent tests and doctors' visits.

When I called her, she said she was fine and wanted to go home. "The food is lousy and they keep sending me for tests." The cardiologist recommended putting her on aspirin, which is also used to decrease the risk of blood clots. It isn't the ideal drug treatment but, at the time, the more recent studies showing the real benefits of Warfarin were not yet in the mainstream medical literature. I reluctantly agreed to his decision and felt that I should not influence my mother against her wishes to take a treatment that had substantial side effects.

Immediately when exiting the hospital parking lot, my mother, eager to leap back into the stream of her activities, insisted on dropping in to visit an ailing relative. "Can you imagine," she recounted to me, "that I caught my foot in the car door and fell and banged my knee! I look like a school kid — all black and blue." What relief I felt that she was not on Warfarin; she would have bled profusely from the fall. It seemed so incongruent that my mother, such a graceful and fluid dancer, had a propensity to fall! This tendency, and her level of activity at her local seniors' centre, put her at high risk for anticoagulant therapy. Her cardiologist's decision appeared to be the right one.

During the next few weeks, each time I spoke to my mother who said she was fine and active and dancing away at the seniors' centre, I felt relieved at the decision that had been made. Then came the distraught call from my father, "Mommy collapsed and I called 911. I couldn't move her from the bathroom — she is in the hospital." She was at a local city hospital, not the HMO (Health Maintenance Organization) hospital where she was previously a patient.

I called my sister Diti (a nickname for Diane) in Chicago and we co-ordinated our flights to New York. The taxi ride from LaGuardia to the house in Brighton Beach was filled with scenes remembered from child-hood as we passed familiar landmarks. We got closer to our house and I recognized the bicycle path where my father took Diti and me for long bike rides when we were youngsters.

The news at the emergency department was shattering. My mother had had a massive left CVA (stroke), leaving her paralyzed down the right side of her body and requiring ventilator-assisted breathing. It was the beginning of the Memorial Day weekend in May with the hospital short-staffed and frenzied and the emergency room a "holding pen" until beds on wards became available. And there lay my mother amidst beds and stretchers of bodies, on a ventilator, suddenly so frail and helpless. I took my father's hand as we approached her bedside. It was impossible to reconcile this scene with the images of my gregarious mother, twirling across the dance floor, with vibrancy and joy. I gazed at her, and in that instant I realized that our lives with my mother would never again be the same. I clung to echoes of her laughter as she would tell a story or watch the antics of my children. I knew that my beloved mother had a tough and uncertain road ahead.

At home my father explained again, "She was in the bathroom, all dressed up getting ready to go to the centre, when I heard a scream and a bang, like something falling. I had trouble pulling her out of the bathroom and used the bathroom rug under her to help move her. I dragged her out of the bathroom but I couldn't get her up. I called 911 and they rushed her to the hospital.

"She hadn't been feeling that well but insisted on going to the centre. I told her she shouldn't go because she might collapse on the way — and then it happened in the house."

In a way it was comforting to know that, up to the very moment she was felled by the stroke, my mother was enjoying her active life.

My mother was moved to a six-bed hospital room, and the nurse reported that she had opened her eyes for a moment a bit earlier, but had not responded to her name. The CAT scan confirmed the stroke, and a program to anticoagulate her was started. I was a bit shocked that she was on a ventilator on a regular medical floor, rather than in ICU (intensive care unit). But the medical resident explained that there were no ICU beds and they thought it was best to move her out of the emergency room. We arranged for private duty nursing to supplement the regular nursing staff, which we could see was inadequate for the task at hand.

I noticed that my mother was on a regular mattress and asked about moving her to a pressure-reducing one. The nurse said, "This is the Memorial Day weekend, and we can't get a pressure-reducing mattress until Tuesday." I was really worried about her developing a pressure ulcer from being immobilized for three days, but she reiterated that there was nothing she could do. She promised that the nurses would shift her position as frequently as they could. The problem seemed to reflect the whole hospital, which was run-down having been built sometime when I was a youngster in the 1950s. Now, like many of New York's city hospitals, it was understaffed and dilapidated..

We all sat around the bed and took turns going out, walking around the hospital floor and going down to the coffee shop, not knowing if Roz was going to survive and, if so, what kind of recovery she would make. By Sunday morning my mother opened her eyes and, with apparent recognition, tried to talk but could not because of the tube in her throat. Her right side was completely paralyzed and her face was drooping, but at least her eyes were opened and she seemed to be able to focus on us and follow our conversation. She indicated that the tube was bothering her. The doctor said he was going to try to remove it and hoped that she could breathe on her own. When the tube came out it was wonderful to see her whole face. She tried to speak, but couldn't because of the stroke. My father left the room and started crying in the corridor. Diti and I held him and told him that we would do whatever it would take to get her better.

The next few months were full of both hope and despair with endless physical and emotional stress as Diti and I alternated or overlapped our visits to Brooklyn. Supporting my father on the phone was not easy; he was despondent. With every small improvement he was hopeful and with every small setback he was devastated. There were moments of humour and pathos, deep drama, and the sharing of basic human emotion with other families whose loved ones shared the various hospital rooms with my mother. One time, soon after the ventilator was removed my mother indicated by scrawling with her left hand that she wanted a cup of coffee or as she would have said in her Brooklynese "cuppa cawfee." My mother loved coffee and it was a joyful step to provide her with a cup, even if it went through the feeding tube. It was only after that tube was finally removed that she was able to drink some coffee very slowly through a straw and enjoy its taste.

My mother played the piano and was an accomplished ballet dancer in her youth and as an adult. She was a devotee of dance and music. As children, even though we did not have a lot of money, my mother made sure Diti and I had music lessons and she often took us to concerts, shows, and ballet performances, which we enjoyed even though we always had the least expensive seats. Those times were special experiences in my life and set the stage for my own lifelong appreciation of music and dance.

I thought that bringing music to her would be therapeutic. We bought a portable tape recorder with earphones and put on Tschaikowsky's Nutcracker Suite. Her face lit up and she started moving her good hand and her head rhythmically to the music. Most poignant was that she started pointing the toe of her left foot, the way a dancer does. We went through tape after tape, my mother responding to music that I knew she loved, Gershwin, Mozart, Beethoven, and one of my favourites, Rachmaninov, whose second piano concerto was one of the first records we ever owned in the family. She kept the earphones on throughout most of the day, and we instructed the privately hired care-givers to keep the music going. It added meaning to my mother's day, and without it she had little to look forward to.

She had some major setbacks; a week after she was admitted a blood clot lodged in her left leg, and Diti struggled to get urgent medical help. Emergency surgery successfully removed the clot and appeared to salvage the leg. It was during that time of post-operative intensive care admission that the most terrible outcome of her hospitalization fully developed: a terrible deep and painful pressure ulcer on the lower part of her backside. During this period, we became very close as a family, dealing with fears and hopes and sleeping again in the very small home that we grew up in. Diti and I strengthened an already great and affectionate respect for each other. It was an unfortunately painful way of enriching our close and loving relationship.

We optimistically welcomed my mother's transfer to the hospital's rehabilitation unit. We began to fantasize that she would go home, and we began to explore what it would take to modify the little house to accommodate her. How would my father, who had significant angina, be able to care for her? We explored how much outside help would be required, but also looked at nursing homes in Brooklyn. Diti investigated nursing homes in her neighbourhood of Oak Park, Illinois, thinking that both my parents could move there. We even enquired into how she could be moved by an air ambulance. At one point my father almost accusingly asked me why I could not get her into the geriatric centre where I worked in Canada. I explained the immigration issues, but because he persisted I looked into it, and was told that we could not take an ill person into the country, even with monetary guarantees, because of the high financial risk to the publicly funded health care system. It was when I was in the process of exploring this option further that my mother's condition suddenly got worse with the development of gangrene in her left, non-paralyzed leg.

When the gangrene was diagnosed the surgeon told us she would need a leg amputation at least above the knee, if not at the hip depending on what transpired. This would mean she would be left with a completely right paralyzed leg and little or no left leg. It was hard for us to imagine that Roz, the person who loved to dance and move to music, would have agreed to such a state of affairs if she had been able to discuss such a choice with us. Since she had her stroke, we could not really communicate effectively with her, but we did the best we could as a loving family who felt we understood her values.

We had arranged for Jessica, a wonderful woman who had looked after another family member for years, to assist in her care and feeding as our HMO would no longer approve private duty nursing. We observed that the unit nurses were too busy to provide adequate care. The knowledge of a loving and caring person being with her for many hours during the evening and night, especially when Diti and I were not in New York, was very comforting.

Then came the ultimate choice. My mother required morphine to quell the pain from her leg that was already gangrenous and from the deep pressure ulcer. Her level of consciousness was variable but through moaning and grimacing when she was awake she indicated that she had terrible pain. Diti, my father, and I struggled with the decision. It was impossible to imagine her living with the expected state of leg paralysis and the amputation. With heart-wrenching effort we decided to decline surgery, but rather treat her with painkillers and let nature take its course. The physician suggested putting in a feeding tube, but we decided that it would prolong her agony and we rejected that as well. The doctor, who had palliative care experience, sympathetically agreed with us, but some of the nurses accepted the decision only reluctantly. One nursing supervisor had the audacity and insensitivity to ask me why I was "starving my mother to death" by not putting in a feeding tube. I had to control my rage when I explained that our family wanted my mother to have as peaceful a death as possible under the circumstances.

I spoke to the doctor, who concurred with our request to treat my mother palliatively, using morphine round the clock as is done with patients dying from cancer. Despite the medical order, it soon became apparent that the nurses kept waiting for my mother to express pain before giving her the injection. Diti or I had to persistently ask, sometimes almost beg, the nurses to give her the morphine at the appointed time, and reiterate that the order read "every four hours round the clock" not "as required," the latter being the usual way of writing non-palliative morphine orders.

The vigil began. My father had the greatest difficulty watching her suffer, and we generally did not leave him alone in her room. Diti or I sat with our mother for hours on end, listening to her rhythmic breathing, with the rasping sound from secretions gathering in her chest. She was not awake and did not seem to hear what we said even though we spoke to her of our love for her. I put the earphones from the tape recorder on my head and turned on Rachmaninov's second piano concerto. That has had a profound affect on me since the first time I heard it in our one bedroom apartment in Brighton Beach when I was about 7 years old. It sustained me through medical school, and now I listened to it over and over again as it wove itself into my mother's laboured breathing.

Exhausted, we decided to go home for the night. Jessica was to stay there to be with Roz. Early in the morning, Jessica called with the news, "Come to the hospital now; it's over." Sadly my mother died with Jessica, rather than with any of her family by her side. Diti and I went to the hospital. She was lying in the bed, uncovered, with an ECG machine connected to her, a last rites ritual of a medical system that seemed to forget dignity but was enthralled with technology. I started pulling out the intravenous line and the nurse began to object. I firmly told her I was a physician and her son and could not bear seeing her in this undignified condition, uncovered and with tubes connected to her. Neither the on-call physician nor any of the nurses uttered a word of condolence. It was just business as usual. We covered her with the sheet and collected the few items from her side table and went to the office to sign the papers. Her ordeal was over. The 10 weeks of coming and going as the long-distance son and daughter was over. Now there was only my father, in the small bungalow that had been our home and now was his alone.

After the funeral and the mourning period, we tried to help my father organize and clean the house. He said he wanted to stay there and assured us that he would be fine. One of us called almost every day. The few friends and neighbours and his sister who lived in Queens tried to lend a hand, but mostly he wanted to be left alone. We knew he was shopping for groceries because the supermarket debits showed up on the credit card, which he shared with Diti. He rejected the idea of rejoining the seniors' centre and claimed he had gone there only to please Roz. We figured the real reason was that he was afraid that he would break down and start crying, something he did whenever he talked about our mother.

Our periodic visits revealed that he was "managing," but the state of the house was deteriorating. He rejected any outside help in cleaning or cooking. We thought he might be depressed, but with time he seemed to express his normal interest in reading his papers, especially the financial sections, and he watched television. He continued to visit some friends from the seniors' centre. but refused to attend any activities despite urging from everyone. He rejected most invitations to join his sister in a meal, but when Diti or I visited he would agree to eat out with us and his sister and her husband and seemed to enjoy himself.

We struggled with his future, even though he said he was fine. I decided to try and get him resident status in Canada. My father agreed to apply acknowledging how much he and Roz enjoyed their frequent visits to Toronto. After the certificate allowing him entry arrived, he said, "I'm not sure I am going to move. Will I have to take a new driving test?" I could not answer for sure, but was pretty certain that he would eventually have to qualify for an Ontario licence. He expressed reluctance to submit to reapplying for a licence, as he was concerned that he might fail the test.

During a visit to Toronto he expressed other doubts. "You know I will probably have to pay more income tax in Canada,." he commented.

"But, you get more in the way of services here" I replied.

"What kind of services do I need?" he asked.

I reminded him of the cost of the long-term care facility that we visited when Roz was sick, and he nodded in agreement. But after the weeklong visit, he was eager to go home, and once there he said he wasn't ready to move. I tried to cajole him, reminding him how hard it was to look after Roz with us being so far away.

"I understand but I can't make the move yet" was his reply. His certificate of immigration expired. He was staying at the bungalow in Brooklyn. Diti and I reluctantly agreed that he had to do it his way.

He occasionally visited me in Toronto or Diti in Chicago. During each visit he seemed a little more frail, but he was still independent in all of his activities. He became increasingly sloppy, but that was always part of his character. We enjoyed his visits and he took pride in seeing his grandchildren and experiencing some of their activities like hockey games and their playing their musical instruments. But he was always eager to return; sometimes he suggested he would cut his usual week-long visit short, only agreeing to stay the full week when I told him the cost of changing his flight.

The house in Brooklyn was looking worse and worse. He tried to fix the bathroom shower faucets, but succeeded in breaking the wall in the process. The float in the toilet broke, and being the engineer, do-it-yourself expert, fixed it by rigging a primitive combination of clips that could be pulled in order to flush. He became embroiled in a lawsuit with a neighbour whose new medical building compromised his ability to use the house's side entrance. That five-year legal case became the focus of all of his psychological energies and most telephone conversations centred around the topic. The case was finally settled out of court, although my father was never satisfied and complained he never had "his day in court."

We visited to celebrate his 89th birthday. Diti arranged a dinner with his sister and her husband. On the way to the restaurant we stopped to buy him a new television as a birthday gift. At dinner, he ate well, but slowly and very tentatively. Afterwards, when he was alone with Diti as the rest of us went to get the car, he turned to her and asked, "How did I get here?" Diti and I took him home and noticed some over-the-counter sleeping medications on his bedside table. Because of a recent episode of low back pain, his physician had given him some strong analgesics.

During this visit, Diti and I noted the dramatic deterioration in my father's functioning. The house was a complete disaster. There were mouse droppings everywhere. We found multiple cheques written for the same bill, each addressed, but not sent out. And we found monthly cheques made out to a charity, but not one that had ever been special to him. It seemed he had forgotten to whom he had sent money. He admitted to falling a couple of times, and recently hit his head and cut his forehead. He blamed it on tripping because of the clutter in the house.

Diti and I agreed that the decision could no longer be left to him. Diti said, "We are moving you to Chicago." We waited for his standard adamant refusal. Instead, he nodded in agreement. Diti told him she would go back to Chicago and see what was available that would provide independence and privacy. He agreed again.

It was now Diti's turn to go through the process of thinking about how and where to move my father. With great luck she found availability in a retirement home five minutes from where she lived. Three weeks later, we both returned to Brooklyn to help him move. The plan was for Diti to drive to Chicago with our father in his small car. We spent a weekend trying to clean up the house, but mainly identifying the papers and personal affects that he would want to take with him. We lined the streets with green garbage bags filled with things we had decided could be tossed.

It wasn't easy to identify essential papers, income tax forms that had not been filed, and bills that hadn't been paid. But gradually things fell into place and Diti and my father were ready to leave. At first, he climbed into the driver's seat saying he would drive because he knew the route better than Diti. I was concerned that he would actually insist on driving, but Diti managed the scene by gently saying, "You can't drive, I need you to navigate." And with that she held his hand to help him out of the driver's side of the car, put him in the other side, and gave him the maps. He seemed satisfied in this role.

That night I received a call from Diti. "What a trip," my sister laughingly said. "First of all it took two hours to get out of New York because although daddy thinks he can navigate and I assumed he could, we got lost a few times before we got on the highway." She continued, "Then the fun began. It was like travelling with a two-year-old just recently potty trained. I drove into every rest stop and insisted that he go to the bathroom. It made for a very long trip. His back was hurting and he really was slow, so I had to pull him out of the car, hold his hand to go to the bathroom, and help him back. He kept asking if I was tired, offering to drive."

I was relieved that they had made it to the halfway mark only a little later than expected. Diti went on, "Daddy thinks this is a pretty swanky motel because it's a cut above the Motel 6 he's used to, although it's not really that fancy. But he thinks its great. He even asked if it has a casino and said if I want some money to gamble he would give it to me." We both roared with laughter.

The next night I spoke to Diti again. "We made it, but it was a trip that was so exhausting I cannot believe I did it". I asked if he recognized the neighbourhood when they drove through it even though he had not been there for some years. "Oh yes. He named the streets and started giving me directions on how to get to the house. He asked about the shops and was surprised when I told him that some of them were no longer in business."

His apartment at the retirement community had been newly painted and carpeted. It was nicely furnished and even had paintings on the walls, and it had a lovely modern kitchen. Diti and I assured him that we would not sell the house unless he wanted to, but that he had to make a minimum five-month commitment to the apartment. Diti asked the home to furnish an extra bed so that she could stay over on a moment's notice, if necessary, which my father liked.

After two weeks, in keeping with my father's independent, stubborn nature, he declared he was ready to go back home to Brooklyn. Diti reminded him that he had agreed to stay five months, and that he would be obligated to pay for the apartment whether or not he stayed.

Diti visited him several times a day during those first weeks to help him acclimatize, often staying with him during the daily luncheon program on his floor. She sat with him and engaged others in conversation to break the ice and help him meet people. She placed his medications in a pillbox to prevent the kinds of mix-ups we suspected had been happening in Brooklyn. When she couldn't visit, she called to do everything to encourage the success of his move.

The township offered a program of discounted meals at local restaurants for seniors. Max loved this program, especially one restaurant that offered good food and ample neighbourhood action. The waitresses began to know him, remembering that he preferred soup, not salad, along with his French fries, chocolate ice cream, and tea. Diti thanked the restaurant owner for helping our father to adjust and see what a wonderful place Oak Park was. Max, a true product of the depression, appreciated being served a $10 meal for $3. He began to say what a nice neighbourhood it was that he now lived in.

One evening he called Diti saying he was feeling really bad. He was having a terrible bout with constipation - something that had plagued him for many years in Brooklyn – and said he needed to go to the hospital. Thinking a trip to the hospital wasn't necessary, Diti instead gave him water, stool softeners, and watermelon as he sat on the toilet. He used glycerine suppositories and finally was successful. Diti stayed overnight on the bed set up for just such a situation. The next day, she was able to challenge his thought that maybe he could go back to Brooklyn. She asked him "What would you have done last night if I hadn't been five minutes away?" He conceded. This was the turning point to his agreeing with the permanency of the move.

Diti knew that he was making a very positive adjustment when he began to relay details of conversations he was having on his own with people in the lunchroom. Sometimes he would read his *New York Times* (the only resident getting this paper delivered) in the lounge rather than going back to his apartment. He always wore a baseball cap that had Indiana written on it, and he found that it provided a nice icebreaker, as people would ask him if he were from Indiana. In his most engaging way he'd say, "No, but I passed through it on my way from New York." Diti was able to lessen her visits to once a day and then occasionally missing a day here or there. He would tell people that Diti had "shanghaied," him and she would retort, "No, I kidnapped him."

After three months in the apartment, he announced he wanted to visit Brooklyn. His decision to move had happened so fast that there were people to whom he hadn't said good-bye. He worried they would wonder why he never answered his telephone.

Diti took him home and they visited the few really special friends he had left behind. He repeatedly described his new living arrangement in Oak Park very positively. At the end of the Brooklyn visit he said, "I am ready to sell the house." We were ecstatic! Fortunately, the next door neighbour was a realtor, and before they returned to Chicago, a contract was signed. My father conceded that life in Oak Park was a much easier and nicer life than he had had in Brooklyn during the previous few years.

One month after the move, his new medical insurance was in place. He had a complete medical examination by a colleague of mine and his medications were modified so that many of the problems that plagued him in Brooklyn, like his back pain, were brought under control. To our delight, with these changes and some additional medications that he needed, his mental state improved remarkably, as did his mood and interactions.

A few more months passed including the Chicago winter, and my father settled in nicely to the retirement home. He gradually began to participate in the various social activities. Each phone call seemed more positive and Diti said he admitted that he had been doing very poorly in Brooklyn and expressed gratitude that we had "forced" him to move. He even said, "You saved my life." I found phone conversations to be like years ago. I could discuss world events and politics. One Sunday evening I asked him about what was in the *Times* and he said, "I don't get the *Times* any more."

I asked with concern, "Why not, are you having trouble reading it?" (This was a man who read the *New York Times* every day of his adult life).

"No" he replied, "I started getting the *Chicago Tribune* instead because it has local news. I thought it was worth knowing what's going on here." To me that was the best indicator that he was staying in Chicago and that his mental function was probably as good as anyone could possibly hope for.

The issue of his driving came up from time to time. We had made a decision to not allow him to drive, and Diti kept his car on her driveway. In reality he had no reason to drive, but as is often the case, he considered not driving as a serious blow to his independence. We understood the impact that the loss of the licence might have for him, so we agreed to look into the Chicago regulations, hoping that with time it would become less and less of an issue. His insurance was changed from New York to Illinois and he saved thousands of dollars with that alone.

We got him new Illinois plates — handicapped ones because of his bad back and angina – but put off applying for a new licence. A couple of times Diti would take him for his favourite drive to the country and find a secluded place and let him drive. After no more than 15 minutes, he was tired and was willing to give up the wheel.

Things were progressing very well with most of the details of my father's health gradually being addressed. One of the outstanding issues was his hearing. He had been resistant to wearing a hearing aid even though it was clear to everyone around him that he had hearing problems. We had modified his phone and encouraged him to seek advice, which he refused. On one of his visits to Toronto I arranged for him to have an excellent hearing evaluation at the Baycrest Centre for Geriatric Care where I work. The audiologist was very perceptive when she responded to his statement that "My hearing is fine, you know." She showed him the audiogram, appealing to his engineering expertise and said to my father, " Mr. Gordon, you are correct that your hearing is okay, but you have major problems with discrimination of sound. Although you might hear the sound, you cannot figure out its meaning." He accepted the explanation, but later on again declined consideration of a hearing aid saying that it was not necessary. In the meanwhile Diti and I struggled with telephone conversations, repeating ourselves many times and speaking slowly when it was clear my father failed to understand what we had told him.

Then in March 2001, on a Friday just prior to my family's winter ski vacation, I received a call from Diti, "Daddy fell this morning in the bathroom, but he seems okay and I am taking him for his scheduled hearing aid assessment." That appointment turned out to be fortuitous. While registering at the local hospital for the assessment, Max had a momentary seizure-like episode. His face grimaced, his left arm went up involuntarily, and Diti screamed for help. He was immediately transferred to the hospital's next door emergency room.

The nurse picked up the phone as my father was being hooked up to the cardiac monitor and said to me, "The tracing looks to me like he is in some kind of heart block." The next day, the cardiologist confirmed that he might need a pacemaker but wanted to observe him further over the weekend to make sure the problem was not related to any of his medications. I assured Diti and my father that should he need a pace-maker the procedure was very safe and effective. By this time my family and I were in Quebec on our holiday. While my wife and children were out skiing, I stayed at the condo and did my writing and reading, staying close to the phone.

The day after the pacemaker was inserted, my father had an episode of vague chest pain, which turned out to be a small heart attack. The medical team at first thought that he could be treated with an angio-plasty (a balloon widening of the heart's blood vessels), but it soon became clear that he would require urgent bypass surgery. I explained the urgency and poor prognosis without surgery to my father over the phone. He said, "Let me think about it."

I replied, "You have about five minutes to think because if it's not done you probably won't be around for very long."

He said, with hardly a moment's hesitation, "Okay, if that's the case."

Surgery was booked for the day we were driving back to Toronto. There was no way I could get to Chicago to be with him, but I spoke to him the night before and I arranged a flight for the next morning. Diti kept me posted during the drive.

Max had indicated to Diti what outcome he would accept from his surgery and what limits he would want on care should it not be suc-cessful. I was very concerned about the possible deleterious effects of major surgery on his mental function, but other than a short period of confusion related to the pain medications, his mind was quite clear. He even started making humorous remarks to the nurses who appeared to thoroughly enjoy him. They were all very impressed with his rapid men-tal and physical recovery. Within the week he was on the rehabilitation unit. Two more weeks and he was sent back to his retirement home. He now knew, for sure, that his move to Oak Park had literally saved his life.

With his 90th birthday coming up, I planned a visit to help celebrate. It coincided with a conference on aging in Chicago, so I took advantage of the opportunity to work and celebrate at the same time. The three of us went out for dinner, and after the meal my father said, "I want to see if after I eat and walk I get chest pain the way I used to." I remember those years when my father would stop before he went for a walk to "catch his breath" and usually take a nitroglycerine pill in order to provide angina relief. We walked up the street and then down and my father said, "I don't feel anything; the surgery really worked." Of course he had not had the surgery because of angina, but because of the small heart attack, but the "side effect" of the surgery was improvement of his angina.

Soon after, an offer came through on the house and Diti and I were confronted with the prospect of actually cleaning the place. We knew that my parents had saved almost everything, so the prospect of making it ready for possession was not pleasant and loomed over us. We had planned to bring my father down to see the house again before we emptied it, but because of his heart surgery we had to cancel that plan. It was, therefore, left to Diti and me to do the job. I suggested that we just hire a dumpster and have the house emptied. Diti, rightfully as I soon learned, disagreed.

It was late Friday night when I arrived. Diti had already packed many bags with clothes and an equal number with garbage, gradually emptying overfilled cupboards and dressers, of which my parents had many. At one point she stopped and asked, "So you want to just throw everything out?" as she handed me my original birth certificate which she had plucked from between some old papers stuffed in one of the dresser drawers. Although I had long ago obtained a copy of it, I held the original in my hand and wondered what other treasures we might find in the little three-bedroom bungalow.

Each item resulted in a comment or observation and some past association was evoked. There was no rhyme or reason to where things had been stored. A box of childhood and family pictures was in one drawer; Diti's grade five school essay was in another; my high school yearbook was in yet another. We found the bill of sale of the Sohmer baby grand piano that our grandmother purchased for our mother in 1935, the one on which I learned to play. We found the receipts of the mother's milk our parents had to purchase after I was born prematurely because I could not tolerate anything else.

We found a letter from our bubbie (grandmother) to our mother, then pregnant with Diti and still in Dearborn, Michigan. It assured her that we could live with her in her Brighton Beach apartment and that my mother needn't wait until my father's transfer from Dearborn where he worked for the U.S. Department of Defense. The letter brought back memories of the apartment we lived in before we moved into the house: the large single bedroom where Diti and I and our bubbie slept, our parents sleeping in the living room with a bookcase separating their "bedroom" area from the rest of the living room, which contained the baby grand piano, a sofa, and some chairs.

The most poignant discovery was a typewritten letter from our mother to her father who had unfortunately abandoned the family to pursue another relationship. The letter pleaded with him to be the father she remembered — when her mother sang opera and he played the English concertina. The letter brought us to tears as we read of the pain she struggled with in trying to come to terms with the problematic relationship she had with her father. It also left us puzzled because our mother had never typed. We wondered who might have helped her write this letter. We couldn't know if it actually was ever sent and we were looking at a copy, or if she had never mailed it to him. It reminded us painfully of the absence of our mother and the many struggles of her life. We could not ask her questions about the letter.

As we found other things, we were grateful that we were doing this job while our father was still alive. Later we could ask him who people were in old photographs or named in documents. I asked about a hospital record we found showing that I had had required a blood transfusion as a premature baby. He confirmed that the blood for the transfusion came directly from him to me – the way all transfusions were done in 1941. The scar at the elbow crease of my left arm from that transfusion has often been the subject of conversation whenever I donated blood.

We found a document required by Max for work that listed all the personal details of immediate relatives, including dates of birth, and city and country of origin. It was a wonderful record of our family history, confirming our Jewish Lithuanian heritage and showing our name, Gordon, had never been changed as so many immigrant names had. As well, this document confirmed the Scottish link to our name, something I had discovered years before while studying in Scotland.

We were very happy to find pictures of our mother in her youth in artistic poses from her ballet and interpretative dancing days. Other pictures much later in her life were of her dancing at the local senior citizens' centre, was such an important focal point of her life. Although she gave up professional dancing aspirations when she got married, throughout her lifetime she and my father would be the subject of much admiration whenever they danced together in public. I recall at my wedding in Winnipeg, to my wife Gilda, how guests remarked to me how wonderfully they danced and especially how expressively and beautifully my mother moved. At the retirement home, my father still was able to take part in the social dances, and Diti has danced with him when he was 90. She recognizes that being able to dance with him is a great gift and part of the legacy from his life with our mother. We slogged along filling bags and showing each other nostalgic finds, always making sure that anything my father might want or need was kept. We called him occasionally to ask if we could throw out some item or other. He asked us to keep some old *New York Time*'s clippings, as he wanted to read them again.

On the second day of our cleanup, Diti yelled from the basement that she found something special and chided me again for having suggested that we just call in a hauling company to take everything. It was two huge boxes of personal letters. It seemed like every letter ever exchanged among us was in these boxes. There were hundreds, including those from my six-month trip to Europe when I was 19 years old and many more from my six years of medical studies in Scotland, my one year as a draft-dodging landed immigrant in Montreal, and my fours years living in Israel. There were letters from the two years that Diti spent in the Peace Corps in Tunisia. There were letters from old friends.

We started reading them, some to each other when we shared the person or the experience, some on our own, because they were very personal.

The letter that caused both Diti and I to laugh most together was one she wrote from summer camp when she was 14 years old. In it, the essence of her intelligence, sensitivity, and maturity came out loud and clear, and within its commentaries and questions was evidence that our relationship was built on and continues to flourish because of the strong values and trust that our parents had in the two of us. Cleaning the house increased the bonds that tie the two of us, and make us realize even more that the legacy of our parents is imprinted indelibly upon us.

Finally, we finished the job, had a few more visits to get the house ready for everything that was headed for the dumpster that was eventually required, and closed the deal. The home of our youth was no longer ours. My father no longer had a place to return to in Brooklyn. Chicago was now his home and at least he had Diti (who I had renamed "Diety") close to him to help him care for himself. I was still the distant son, trying to be of assistance by phone and the occasional visit and through very close communication with Diti. She has assumed the major part of caregiving. She has done it all with the greatest love and devotion that anyone could ever expect from a child. We have concluded that it is all part of being a caring and loving family and that there really could and should not be any other way, although we know that many times things do not work out so well in families.

My father has come through a lot. Now we just take one day at a time and enjoy the fact that he has a life with a lot of interests and satisfactions and that we are able to still enjoy his presence, his humour, and his still sweet and engaging personality.

Lessons learned

The experiences I had with my mother has taught me a number of lessons that I have been able to use in helping my father, and from my experiences with both of them, I have learned lessons that have helped me in my clinical geriatric practice. I can now understand the predicaments of patients and their families not only from the professional perspective, but from the personal vantage as well.

From the experiences with my mother, I learned it was important to do some talking earlier, rather than later. I have done my best to make sure that I know my father's values and wishes should he fall seriously ill and not be able to make decisions. I realized that sitting down and putting together a written living will was not going to happen. Therefore I told him what I thought the important values were in his life and how I would make decisions if he were to become ill in a manner similar to my mother. When he confirmed these values and principles, I communicated them to my sister. This proved to be very useful when it came time for his cardiac surgery. All he had to do was say that he wanted to be "left alone" if he did not make a good recovery, and that was enough for us to understand what he meant by this statement.

I also learned from my mother's illness that children often find it difficult to accept bad outcomes and often take it upon themselves to try and rectify the situation, especially in institutional settings. This reaction is reasonable and when done properly can lead to some improvements in care. It is useful to understand what clinical options make sense and try to act on them. It is important to not allow others to make decisions for you. Well-meaning people may provide advice and input, but ultimately it is the family that has to decide what is "right." However, once that decision is made, it is important not to question it. I use this concept with my patients and families who struggle with decisions. I try and help them understand that there are rarely "right" answers to difficult decisions, and they can only do the best they can and must live with their decision, knowing it was the best one they could have made under the circumstances.

A lesson I learned from caring for my father is knowing that timing is often critical in decision-making. It is not possible or necessarily proper to force a situation on a parent if he or she is not ready for that decision to be made. It is counterproductive to badger your parents into making a decision that they are not yet prepared for. I learned this when my father was reluctant to move from his home — until it was clear that he was in danger. And I learned it again when he refused a hearing aid; when he was ready, that was the only time to act. On the other hand, I also learned that sometimes waiting until someone is "ready" may be too late and too dangerous. I try and help patients and their families make difficult decisions by outlining the implications of waiting too long to make a necessary move.

Another important lesson I have learned is that you *can* teach an "old dog new tricks." The opportunities to grow and develop can continue at every age. Moving out of the family home into a a "facility" does not have to be the beginning of the end. Rather it may be the beginning of a new era of interaction and enjoyment. I have seen this in my practice, but most important I have now experienced it with my father. He has been transformed from an almost hermit-like existence, deteriorating physically and mentally, to a vibrant, active person who participates in social activities including dancing and exercise pro-grams. To see him greeted by his "buddies" at the retirement home lunch program is very satisfying for me as I know that once again my father Max is a "somebody."

The last and perhaps most important lesson I've learned is that as a child, helping your parents can be very challenging, trying, and time-consuming. If possible, try and share the responsibility with other sib-lings, and if that is not possible, at least acknowledge and support the sib-lings that are carrying the main part of the responsibility. I am lucky to have a wonderful sister who is the primary caregiver to my father. I must remind myself how fortunate my father and I are to have my sister. On the other hand, both my sister and I were fortunate to have had our par-ents, and caring for them in their later years is a small way of returning to them the wonderful lives that they were able to provide for us and the values that they instilled in us.

Update:
A Week of Trauma Turns Our Lives Upside Down
by
Bart Mindszenthy

I FINISHED DRAFTING THE INTRODUCTION TO this book on April 20. Now, only three months later, we're into a new family crisis.

When I started work on *Parenting Your Parents* and Michael Gordon agreed to join with me on this journey, it was my father who was ill and in hospital. The problem? Severe constipation. So severe that I had to get him into the emergency room at North York General Hospital twice — first for a not too successful "extraction," which is a very messy form of "digital digging" into his rectum, and then again for enemas and more digital work.

The second round meant staying in the hospital for three days to ensure his bowel was functioning. Plus, my father needed a catheter inserted into his penis because his bladder was blocked. With all this, he was grumpy, miserable, in pain, and "out of it" because of the Demerol injections given to relieve the pain. But with his usual will and tenacity, and because he is willing to listen to what needs to be done, he's regained a bit of his health. He's not in great shape, but he keeps pushing along, every so slowly, and ever so carefully.

Since his hospitalization, my mother has taken a turn for the worse. It's a situation that's been brewing for some weeks. My mother's been like a pot of water on the stove with the heat turned up high — eventually the water boils and if the pot isn't taken off, the water bubbles over. And my mother's mind is now boiling.

What follows is a chronicle of the past week. It's self-explanatory. It's all about what happens when a parent is undergoing rapidly advancing dementia that is suspected to be the dreaded Alzheimer's disease. There's nothing nice about any of this. It's painful for all involved, and right now I feel a huge amount of love for both my mother, who's entering the "twilight zone" of her older age, and my father, who will have to witness his wife of nearly six decades change before his non-seeing eyes into someone who will become totally different in the time they have left together.

If there is a hope, it's that in some way we'll manage to work through this dire challenge and be able to help and support my mother; to make her as comfortable as possible, and to somehow let her know how much we love her and care about her well-being. And it's hoped that my father will be able to cope with the fact that we can't ever go back to where we were: that nothing will be sure or safe or right again in the times ahead.

July 24, 2001

Dementia, my parents' doctor tells me, cuts a broad swath throughout the mind and behaviour of the elderly. Dementia is a single word that means so little and affects so much. It ranges across a spectrum that goes from pre-dementia, to mild, then moderate, through to severe, and then the end stage. Bottom line: cognitive capabilities decline —memory, judgment, insight, and reason. Which is a nice way of saying that the mind is not able to do the work it once did years ago, and that step by step there is a new mindset that is confusing, difficult to accept, and eventually impossible to understand for all those who are in the midst of it.

Dementia means many different things to many people, but what it means most to all of us who have a parent experiencing it, is that there is a growing gap between what we used to experience with a parent, and what is now happening.

My parents' doctor has given my mother a carefully balanced set of medications to help her cope with her increasingly fragile mental state.

She's been tested in just about every imaginable way. A geriatric assessment team has spent time with her twice in the past six months, and then there were the CAT scans and the blood work, and neurologist's examination. All of it has resulted in little more than the conclusion that my mother is far more demented than she was 6 or 12 months ago, and that, in fact, she's now delusional.

This diagnosis is borne out by her most recent allegations that my father — nearing 96 — and one of the women who come in to help them (who's in her late thirties) are having a sexual relationship. The accusations started several weeks ago when my mother became agitated because the helper was stroking my father's arm, and it built from there. Yesterday, my mother claimed that the helper was in bed with my father. Just today, she maintained that the helper was nude in my father's room, then in bed with him. She also asserted that the helper was stealing things from the house and lying about what medication my mother is taking. This afternoon, my mother actually physically attacked my father, hitting and slapping him, and tried to hit the helper with her cane.

I talked to my parents at least a dozen times today on the telephone, because I'm away. The concern, worry, agony, fear, anger, and love are overwhelming as the stress of the situation courses through me. Each time we talk, I hear the beleaguered voice of my father, weak as it is, straining to be heard, telling me how concerned he is about my mother and how terrible he feels — how her imagination is getting the best of her. He asks how I can help, and I tell him that I just don't know, because I'm way beyond my competency given the situation. He wants to me to drive to their house in Toronto, and I ask what that will achieve, and he tells me, probably nothing.

When my mother gets on the phone, she's full of venom. Her anger is awesome and overwhelming. She verbally attacks my father: how could he have sexual relations with this woman after so many years of marriage, all through which she's been faithful and so caring of him and me. And how can he deny his transgression?

And then my mother sets in on me: how is it possible that I, her son, could possibly question her about what she's seen. How is it possible that I would doubt her word when she's always been there for me over these many years. It's a nasty conversation during which I sometimes lose control and verbally shoot back; and sometimes I try very hard to give her comfort.

The reason we have so many telephone sessions is that my mother keeps hanging up on me. Between one such set of calls, I telephone my parents' doctor and leave a message, asking him to call me as soon as he can. Then, in the next call to my mother, she tells me that I've abandoned her, that I've sided with my father, that I've been brainwashed by others, and that I've fallen to the charms of this helper of theirs as well. Along the way, my mother hurls a host of personal insults that sting and tear into my own mind, to a point where I don't know what to do to help my parents or myself.

Somewhere through these conversations, their doctor returns my call and I can hear in his voice the concern for both my mother and my father. He does something very special: he tells me he's going to call my mother tonight to talk with her. And he's going to look at whether it might be best to get her admitted into our local hospital's geriatric ward for a break and an assessment.

Later tonight, I talk on the phone again to my parents. My mother is totally illogical. I try very hard to cope and find some common ground with her. My father sounds even weaker than usual and totally drained, telling me that my mother's mind is confused and that we need to help her. While I agree with him, I don't know what to do or how to do it best. Rushing through my own mind is a mix of frustration, love, and doubt.

They're old, I tell myself. Very old. What can I do for either and both of them? Then my mother comes on the line, still passionate with her anger and hurt. I try very hard to be calm and cool and loving, and it's a challenge as she again rips into me for being selfish and siding with my father and completely blinded by my hate for her.

I don't know how to handle this. My own personal world is in chaos. On the one hand, I want to reach out and hug my mother and remind her that I'm her son and love her and that I'll take care of her forever. On the other hand, I want to yell at her that she's not dealing with the real world and that her mind's playing tricks on her, pushing her further and further into a false world created by her advancing dementia. But I've learned enough working on this book to know that right now challenging her is wrong and of no use. My mother is off into another dimension and the best I can do is try to listen, absorb the hurt, and see if I can in some way generate a calming effect in her. And I fail at this. I'm into new territory I don't know how to manage.

Later that evening, my partner, Gail, provides an excellent reality check by asking me a series of questions over a subdued dinner.

> What do I think I can really do for my mother by being logical when she's not? When did my mother begin to show signs of behaving this way? What did my father or I do help her in the past? How much of this load do I think I can carry, and for how long? How long do I think my parents can manage this family crisis?

The truth is, I don't know the answers to any of Gail's questions. What I do know is that I'm mentally and emotionally and physically drained by what's happened this long day. Late into the night, I'm conscious and worried about my mother and my father, hoping that both can and will sleep deep and well into tomorrow so that we might move on and get this mess behind us.

July 25, 2001

During the night, my mother stayed in my father's bed and talked all night. Once she hit him again, and another helper who stays the night with them tried to restrain her. The helper tells me that both of them are exhausted, yet my mother continues to verbally badger my father, like a tape running over and over again. I hear this when she calls to tell me I'd better come to help. We're staying at our country home for a few weeks, with me going into town every couple of days to check on them, shop for food they need, and get our mail. Gail also stopped by when she was in town last week.

So I rush to the city, and in the process manage to get a hefty speeding ticket. En route I try to call my parents' geriatric specialist, but can't get through. I leave an urgent message, which is never returned. Then I call their family doctor, who calls back quickly. I tell him what's happened and that my mother has also apparently stopped taking her pills; it seems she's claiming that she doesn't know what she's taking or why, and so she's not taking anything. He urges me to bring her into the hospital —where he'll be later in the day — and says that it would be good idea to keep her in for a couple of days to do assessments and get her on her medication. Plus, he says, this would give my father a rest. He also tells me that if I can't get her to come with me, I might have to ask for assistance from the police.

When I get to my parents' house, my mother is still going on about my father and his alleged infidelity. She then takes some well-aimed verbal shots at me. I ask her several times to come with me to the hospital, and she refuses. It's exasperating. Then, suddenly, she agrees to come. She dresses, and then when she's ready and eating their usual very late breakfast, she tells me she's not coming after all — that there's nothing wrong with her if people would just leave her alone. Throughout, she keeps talking in a totally disjointed way — zigging this way and then zagging that way in her train of thought.

And there's a new behaviour I notice for the first time: every time I look at my father, or if I go and do something in another room, or I touch something that's hers, my mother immediately wants to know what I'm doing and if I'm taking something that's hers. Repeatedly she talks about people stealing things from her or from their house. She alleges that we're all in collusion against her. And, worst for me to hear, she tells me over and over that I'm a total disappointment because I'm working against her, believing others and not her. My mother demands to know how I could have changed so much for the worse and who is influencing me to turn against her.

And on and on it goes. And like playing spin the bottle or the roulette wheel, where it stops, no one knows. But it doesn't stop at all. It just changes directions, her mind obviously churning myriad confused thoughts.

On the front porch of their house, where my mother can't hear us, I ask my father what he would like me to do, because it's clear that there's no way she'll voluntarily come with me to the hospital. We discuss options, and I tell him of my concern for both his well-being and hers. He thinks about it, then says that calling the police to take her to the hospital would probably do more immediate harm than if we tried to get her to a calmer state for a day or two and then try again. I'm not convinced. I ask him again to consider the pressure on him, and all of us. But he's thought about it and stands by his decision.

I acquiesce only because I do respect his mind, and because he is a psychologist by training. I know he's old, but my father is mentally strong, even if physically very weak.

When we go back in, my mother asks if my father and I remember that awhile ago we all stood in the hallway, made the peace sign, and shook hands to agree that we'll all be all right again. I reply that didn't happen at all. My father agrees with me. And my mother immediately starts on another harangue about how we're conspiring to work against her. A thought flashes through my mind —something Michael told me in one of our early meetings. He'd said that sometimes, when an older person is demented and delusional, if she or he believes something that's not harmful but neither is it real, it may be all right to let it be real. So I backtrack and tell my mother I don't mean it didn't happen, that I just don't remember. And I propel my father into the kitchen and whisper to him that he should remember we shook hands and agreed, which is precisely what he does as he walks back into the living room. My mother looks victorious; she tells me that this is a good example of my own forgetfulness and confusion. We got a tiny step ahead for the moment, although it wasn't easy.

Moments later, she starts again about why and how I'm not being supportive of her. I manage to inject into her newest outpouring of confused thoughts that I've got some errands to do and that I'll be back later.

So I leave them for a few hours, to get our mail, stop for a brief meeting, and do some grocery shopping for them. Along the way, my 23-year-old daughter, Andrea, calls me on the cell phone, wanting to know how I am and how her grandparents are, and to tell me about what she's doing. I give her a fast update. She's shaken by her grandmother's decline and says she's going to call them and then call me back.

Andrea calls me back some 10 minutes later to report that her grandmother indeed sounds very confused. She tells me that she's very worried by what she's heard, and scared by what her grandmother said, which was, in essence that things are not right and that I'm one of the main causes. Andrea also talked to her grandfather and told him she understands how traumatic this is for all of them, especially for him. Andrea, by the way, is in her final year at university studying neuropsychology. She asks if she should come to help. I'm moved and thank her, but recommend that there's nothing she can do to help right now.

When I return from errands and shopping, my parents are having supper. My mother tells me that while I was away, she and my father had a good talk and that they've agreed to put all this behind them, not talk about it any more, and get on with their lives. I'm delighted, relieved, and hopeful that perhaps we might have gotten over this family crisis. I have a bit to eat with them. Then my mother says we need to have a discussion about how I feel. I tell her that there's nothing to discuss; if they've agreed to put "this" behind them, that's all I care about. I suggest that we should never talk about it again, but it's clear my mother wants to do just that.

By now I'm tired and thinking about the drive ahead. So I tell her that I'm concerned for both of them, and that for the sake of all of us, we should agree not to talk about this any more.

We all agree, and I leave.

And so another intense episode passes. Where this leads, I don't know. I only know I'm very tired. I know I'm watching and experiencing another level of descent into the vortex of dementia and all the challenges it's presenting. How we'll deal with it is a mystery to me. What I do know is that I'm afraid for both my mother and my father — for what each must cope with while we find a way forward and for the strength they will need to face the next hurdle.

July 26, 2001

The phone rings early afternoon. In his strained, reedy voice, my father tells me my mother is again on a verbal binge. She's still stuck in the "how-could-you-do-this-to-me" mode, and he asks me to come back from the country where I'm working on this book to help. I honestly don't want to. I'm terrified of where this is leading.

I can hear my mother in the background yelling at my father to give her the phone, and when he keeps talking to me, I hear her attack him.

It's terrifying. She comes on the line and continues her rant about my father's infidelity about how I don't seem to care, and about her personal hurt and shame. This goes on for a few minutes, and then my father is back on, asking when I can be there. Although I had dedicated this day to writing, I tell him I'll come as soon as possible, but I need to try to reach their family physician first. I try, but he's not in. I call the geriatric clinic and talk to one of the staff who a month ago spent time with my parents in their home. She's very understanding and gives me some good options for getting immediate help. The best is to contact something called the Mobile Crisis Team, and that's what I do first.

The woman who answers the phone at the Mobile Crisis Team is wonderful, understanding, and ready to help once I explain the state of affairs. Heidi tells me a team can be at my parents' house when I get there, and that if they determine there is danger to my mother or father, then they'd arrange to have my mother taken to the hospital, even if it meant calling in the police. I call to tell my father I'm on my way, then I change, jump in the car, and head off.

When I'm about half an hour away from my parents', I call Heidi back. This time I get her partner, Leslie, who explains that they're on the way to another emergency visit, but to call when I get to my parents' house, and that they'll come as soon as possible.

I get to my parents' house, and call Heidi and Leslie on the cell phone while sitting in the car in the driveway. They're busy helping someone else, but they tell me that as soon as they're done — and they're not too far away — they'll come to see us.

I take a deep breath and knock on my parents' front door. My father opens it, looking gaunt and drained. My mother is sitting in her usual chair in the living room. When she sees me, she begins to intensely explain all the wrongs done to her by this conspiracy of people. We talk, argue, back off, start talking some more, and keep going in circles that leave none of us feeling any better. This goes on for an hour.

We continue at the kitchen table while we eat dinner. Then my cell phone rings: it's Leslie to say they're out in front of the house, and I tell them they're needed. When they come in, Heidi takes the lead and she's wonderful: relaxed, easygoing, and non-confrontational. My mother, who for some time has been so vocal and emotional, suddenly is the epitome of sweetness and reason. I'm amazed by this transition. Meanwhile, Heidi just keeps talking and asking questions, and each time my mother gets her back up, Heidi backs down to give my mother more comfort space. For example, when Heidi first asks about what medications she's taking, my mother won't tell, yet five minutes later, she's showing Heidi all her bottles of pills. So it goes for the better part of half an hour, until Heidi asks my mother a series of questions that somehow gets my mother to drop the façade and revert to her behaviour of the past weeks. She becomes more belligerent and aggressive, and keeps questioning why anyone would possibly want to doubt her version of reality.

After also asking my father some questions, Heidi thanks my parents for their time and says goodbye and signals me to follow her out, where, on the front porch, Leslie is concluding a cell phone conversation with another family in distress. As we stand in the driveway, Heidi tells me they can't call the police or anyone else to take my mother into the hospital, because while they believe my mother is delusional and a danger to herself and my father — and even me — there's no observed behaviour to support that contention.

So they give me more options. One is to have my parents' family doctor make a house call and convince my mother to go into the hospital for an assessment. The second is to go to a justice of the peace and plead my case for a ruling that would allow my mother to be forcefully taken to a hospital for an assessment and treatment plan. And, the third is to get a my parents' family doctor or the geriatric specialist to sign a "Form One," and admit her to the geriatric psychiatric section at the local hospital for 72 hours of assessment and treatment.

Some choices. I don't want any of them. Each is plagued with personal and family danger. This is not where I want to be. No matter what I do, I realize, I'm going to hurt someone — my mother, my father, me, my children, my partner, my parents' few remaining friends — which means that as far as my mother is concerned, I'm going to be the villain. That's a lot of weight to carry, I think. But then again, I realize that it's not like I have many workable choices As my friend and colleague Harvey Silver, an organizational psychologist, likes to remind one and all, we always have choices; we just need to consider them and decide, since even doing nothing is a choice we make.

When I go back in to talk to my parents again, I convince my mother to to see the geriatric specialist, whom they'd seen some six months ago. I ask her if she'd come with me to see him so we can talk about what medications she should be taking and to review how she's doing. My mother says she'll come as long as we can also go have a cappuccino together afterward, and I agree. I feel like a traitor, a Judas, because I've already arranged the appointment with the doctor, and I know he'll give her two choices: to voluntarily go straight to the hospital or to have them sign a Form One and have her taken in.

It's on that note that I head for my house in the city to get some sleep. I'm depressed, tired, and confused; I tell myself I'm doing the right thing, and then second guess myself the next moment. I have this ongoing debate in my head about what to do, and recognize that in this case, I simply must get her the kind of help she needs, because we're all self-destructing the way things are going.

July 27, 2001

I call the doctor's office in the morning and talk with the woman who's been my contact and who's met my parents. We discuss the options again, and she assures me that, given her own assessment of my parents about a month ago, we must get my mother into the hospital.

I call my mother and tell her she has to get up and get ready for a 10:45 a.m. session with the doctor, and that she should bring all her medications. Then I get ready, drive to my parents' home and collect my mother and her five bottles of pills. She's agitated, confused, and confusing.

The doctor's office is only a five-minute drive, and we get there on time, and then — what else is new? — we wait. He's running behind. Eventually, he comes to get us and take us to his office. He's not the epitome of warmth and charisma, but he's very good at what he does. So it's a tense meeting right from the get-go. He spends some minutes looking at what's now become a rather thick file, and asks her some questions, many of which my mother doesn't understand; some, neither do I, but I translate as best I can.

The long and short of it is that the doctor asks her to voluntarily check into the hospital immediately. My mother tells him there's nothing wrong with her, and that, no, she won't do that. Then he tells her that if she won't agree to go with me to the hospital, he'll have to sign the Form One and have the police take her there. My mother is clearly devastated, but says, no, she won't go. She looks at me and asks how I could do this to her — her only child, turning on her like this. And on it goes for another five minutes, when the doctor asks us to wait in the reception area.

My mother and I sit there, and for the better part of an hour she assaults me with a host of allegations about my memory, my behaviour, my lifestyle, and everything else she can think of. Added to it all are various threats about what she'll do to me and my reputation and threats about how my father will die if I go through with this. She argues, she pleads, and she verbally attacks me as we sit there; she stops people walking by and asks for help, and she eventually says she wants nothing to do with me ever again and gets up and moves four seats away from me.

I'm in a living real-time hell — as I know she must be. I keep telling her this is not something I want to see happen, or like, but that there just isn't any other choice. We argue, and we ignore each other.

Finally, a squad car with two police officers arrives. They walk over to us and talk with my mother, asking her to come with them. She says she won't. But they are very gentle and caring and amazingly patient. They kid with her, and they compliment her, and they eventually get her to stand up and head for the door. Meanwhile, several staff people are looking on, and some of them even come by and whisper to me that I mustn't take this personally and that I'm doing the right thing.

I'm almost in tears. This is so hurtful and painful. It's real and happening, and it shouldn't be. I feel a huge amount of love and sorrow and anxiety and hurt. It's like the morning my marriage died and I watched the faces of my children as I left. It's one of those experiences that stays with us for a lifetime. All I know is that I don't want to be here, to be in this scene. However, it's still better happening this way, here, not in my parents' home, with my father there.

The police officers are considerate yet again. They suggest that my mother ride in my car, rather than in the patrol car. My mother tells them I'm not her son anymore, and she doesn't care. But in the end, she sits in the front seat beside me, with an officer in the back seat, and the other in the patrol car following. While my mother tells me that I'm the bane of her life and a worthless son she never wants to see again, I, for some crazy reason, become very conscious of driving right at the speed limit and using my turn signal at every turn we make. And so we get to the hospital emergency room, which is flooded with people.

While the officers help my mother check in, I rush back to my parents' house to tell my father what is happening. He sits in stunned, sad silence. He sighs deeply several times. His quivering hands are clutched together, and he looks at me with such sorrow that I want to cry again. I ask him: what else could we do? I ask him: isn't this going to help my mother — his wife of 58 years — get the help she needs? Won't this give him a break from the tension that's been hanging smog-like in their house for the past weeks? My father acknowledges that it's the right thing, but says it hurts, and I see the quiver of his lips for the first time in my life. And I know how much pain he also is experiencing at this moment. He wants to know how long she'll be in the hospital, and I tell him I don't know, even though I do know it's at least four days. But I don't want to make him feel even worse. I keep telling him that it's for the best, and he just nods and tells me that's probably right.

I rush back to the emergency room reception area, and there we wait for two hours. The police officers are helpful and considerate beyond anything I'd have expected. Finally, my mother's name is called, and we're taken to a cubicle in the treatment area. That's where we'll spend the next six hours, locked in verbal combat. I don't want to argue; I keep telling my mother that we're here to get her the help she needs, and she keeps telling me that she's fine. We go around and around in circles of complex and confusing dialogue. A few times I manage to get out and call my father to give him an update, and to call my partner, Gail, to tell her what's going on.

My mother has now decided that this is a jail or prison of some kind. I keep assuring her it's not. And just to add to the drama and trauma of this event, the police arrive with a stocky, barrel-chested man in leg shackles and handcuffs, who's plunked on a bed two cubicles down from where we're sitting. Of course, this adds more fuel to my mother's mental fire. Now we are in a prison, and we're just waiting for her cell to be cleared. And so it goes. We talk nicely, we talk passionately, and we argue. A woman who's been there for almost 24 hours with her aging ill mother waiting for a bed comes by and we strike up a conversation, and this gives me a chance to run out and find a sandwich and juice for my mother and me to share.

Time passes. Finally, two women arrive. They introduce themselves, and I can't remember the name of either. They tell us they're the crisis team. They sit and talk with my mother for about three-quarters of an hour, asking her a lot of questions. My mother responds and does quite well with her broken English. I urge her to tell them what she's most upset about, and she does: about my father's affair with the their helper, and what a shame this is, and how terrible it all is, and how she's over that now, but how it hurts. The two women thank my mother for her time and tell her that soon she'll be moved upstairs.

Then we're alone again for another hour. My mother gives me several ultimatums that are essentially the same: get her out of here and take her home so she can care for my father, or he'll probably die.

Yet another hour passes and finally a cheerful orderly arrives with a wheelchair, only to discover we've already got one. So he picks ours and helps my mother into it, while she continues to tell me I've got one final chance to repent and relent and take her home. I keep telling her that I can't do anything right now and that we've got to get her the help she needs.

Upstairs, on the seventh floor, we are buzzed into the geriatric psychiatry wing. I read the sign, and I watch the procedure, and I'm on the edge of tears again. I can't believe I'm doing this: that my mother is here and so am I.

A bubbly nurse emerges from the locked nursing station and we wheel my mother into a private room with a large glass window in the door and it's own bathroom. Then we tour the self-contained area while some woman with an accent almost as good as my mother's sings in a loud voice somewhere down the hall. By the time we get to the communal dining room, hearing yet a few other people yelling and seeing others walking up and down the hallway, I keep thinking about the book and amazing movie, *One Flew Over the Cuckoo's Nest*. I just can't believe we're here, or that we have to be here. There is something totally terrifying about this, and yet I honestly believe that if we're to save my parents' lives for a while longer, this is what we must do.

Back my mother's room — her cell, as she calls it. I try to get her as comfortable as possible. She's cold, and we get some extra covers, but the fact is hospitals are cold all of the time, and for the elderly this is another discomfort.

I tell her I'll bring some her a bathrobe, some other clothes, and her toiletries. This is of small consolation to my mother. She wants to know again why I did this to her, and how long she has to stay in this terrible place, which, I must admit, it is. She reminds me that I betrayed her and pledges that she won't last more than a day here. She says again that by doing this to her I'm killing her and my father, who can't last on his own.

There's not much I can say. I'm hurting. I feel guilty. I'm tired. I'm scared. I'm 55 years old and would much rather crawl in my mother's arms so we can just hug each other. Instead, I help her change into hospital garb and get her into the bed, and I assure her I'll be back in the morning. I leave, and I want to die of fear and shame.

I go back to my parents' house and sit in the kitchen with my father who's nursing a Scotch and looking so pale and so sad that I don't know what to do or say. We sit there awhile in silence, and I start telling him that things will be all right. I see that he's about to cry — this father of mine who's close to 96 years of age and who's always managed his emotions with perfection. Finally, he agrees that my mother needs the attention and care she'll get at the hospital. He tells me that he knows this is right, but that it's still so very traumatic.

We sit there at the kitchen table and chat for a while. He's also very tired. I go and find a small suitcase and pack up clothes and toiletries for my mother, and when I'm done, I tell him to get some sleep. We agree I'll go see her in the morning and take him in to see her in the early afternoon.

And so we hug and part and I drive to the house in the city, feeling totally empty inside.

July 28, 2001

I get to the hospital late morning after a restless night of sleep. I'm tired and stressed. I'm afraid of what condition my mother will be in when I get there. En route, I stop to buy her a sweat suit, which I think will be comfortable and warm. I buy myself a muffin in the hospital lobby because I'm very hungry. And up I go — back to that seventh-floor "prison."

I buzz. I'm admitted. I go the nursing station and meet and talk with the nurse who's looking after my mother who is very nice and helpful. When she looks at what I have brought, she tells me I can't give my mother any nightgowns, only the bathrobes. I can't give her the sweat suit, but I can give her the toiletries kit, and yes, I was smart to take out the razor blades and substitute one of my electric shavers. She says that my mother's doing all right, but that she's somewhat delusional.

My mother is sitting on the bed. She wants to know if I've come to take her home. No, I tell her, not yet, because they have to do some tests. She gets angry. She wants to know why more tests are needed. She says that she's peeing and pooping quite well, and she wants to go home. And, she tells me, a doctor came in to see her and talk with her and he also said she was doing really well. I show her what I have brought — the bathrobes, socks, toiletries, slippers, and a few other things. Meanwhile, I dig out the muffin and share it with her, while I listen to her tell me what a horrible night she's had.

We spend an hour talking, with my mother seeming more subdued but still very angry with me. I help her into the bathroom and onto the toilet and wait outside until she's done, and then help her get organized again and into a chair when her lunch arrives. Then she starts again to verbally attack me for what I've done to her, and my personal guilt monitor soars at once. While I feel huge pity for my mother, concurrently there is also a sense of anger for these continuing attacks, and I try very hard to control my emotions and my tongue so I don't say something I'll regret and in the process exacerbate an already fragile situation. So I tell her I'm going to get my father to bring him for a visit.

When I wheel him into her room an hour later, she's instantly in tears. He slowly gets out of the wheelchair and she slowly stands, and they hug and kiss. It's both heartwarming and heartbreaking to watch.

I stay a bit, leave them to run some errands. When I return, they're sitting talking as quietly as is possible for people who are hard of hearing. We all chat a while longer and I can see my father is tiring, so I suggest we leave. There are a lot more tears and hugs and kisses before I wheel him back to the car and drive him home, and head back to the country myself.

I'm really, truly tired, both physically and mentally. I've been dashing to their home most days for several weeks, and always spending way more time than I'd anticipated. I'm behind in my client work. And I'm way behind on my parts of this book. Michael is being highly understanding and supportive because he knows what I'm going through on both the personal and professional level. However, I need to get my mind in gear, and it's difficult.

Tonight, I call my daughter Andrea and ask her and her wonderful partner if they'd give me a day off and go see my father tomorrow and take him to visit my mother. They say they're pleased to do so, and that relieves me.

July 29, 2001

It's amazing how tired I am. I worked for a couple of hours on this chronicle of events last night and then fell into bed and woke up not long before noon. I walk around, numb and dumb, for an hour and decide that today for a few hours I need to do mindless work around the property, so I paint things and glue things, and change some light fixtures, and move slowly. I even have a short nap late in the afternoon.

Through it all, I am mulling over the events of the past days, relating them to the past months, and trying to fit those all into the past years. I try to figure out if there is a pattern we missed, or if there is some special event that may be important. I think there are some pieces that loosely fit, but I realize that I'm just speculating.

Then my father calls to say he, Andrea, and Julian had a good visit with my mother, and she seems much calmer over all, and that he misses her and would like her back at home. He also asks me to call her, which I was planning on doing anyway, and see what I think. Then my daughter calls to tell me that her grandmother was in pretty good shape from all she could see and hear. This is heartening news.

I call the geriatric psychiatry wing nursing station and ask how I can speak to my mother. There is one patient phone and it's busy, so the nurse takes pity on me and gets my mother to her phone so we can talk for a few minutes. She actually does sound much more subdued and generally calmer. I feel good about that, although part of me is worried that this may be just a false positive signal and that more bad things may come sooner than later. But even given that cautionary thought, I want to believe that we're on the path to some kind of stable footing for the good of all of us.

July 30, 2001

Early this afternoon, my mother's in-hospital doctor calls. He asks me several questions about how I see her state of mind and general condition now compared to last week, and suggests we meet tomorrow morning. He tells me that he thinks she might be able to go home the next day or so.

I call my father with this news, and I can just sense him perking up right over the phone line. I ask him to think about what's best for him and for her and tell him I'll pick him up in a few hours.

Driving into the city, I reflect on the complexity of being a family member dealing with a loved one who's demented. It's sort of like a Catch-22. If my mother thinks that something that isn't real is real, how do we deal with that? My experience so far is that it's a no-win debate. The people who are watching her witness all sorts of things she's imagined in her mind. There are myriad instances when my mother simply denies reality and clings with a passion to her point of view. My father and I have talked about this many times the past months, and he just shakes his head and tells me sometimes we simply have to let go and let her reality be the one we go with. This troubles me greatly. Where do you draw the line? How do we help our parents find the truth so we can deal with it? Yet as Michael has said to me, sometimes if the reality of a demented person isn't hurtful, maybe it's best to let it be; to let it be their reality. If a demented person with Alzheimer's believes it's Tuesday, for example, but really it's Wednesday, and in the greater scheme of life that doesn't matter, then perhaps that's how we should leave it. I see the sense in all of this, but it's still hard to practice.

By the time I think about all this and end up nowhere, I'm at my parents' house to take my father to see my mother. Today she's sitting in her chair in her room, and she lights up like a birthday candle when I wheel him in. The hugs and kisses are sincere and laden with overwhelming affection. Again, I sit around and talk for a little while and then leave to let them have time alone. And again, when I return, my mother tells me that there's nothing wrong with her mind and demands to know why I am subjecting her to this humiliation and personal pain. Even as she says this, she's confusing things, and alleging things that just aren't so. But it is evident that she is much calmer overall, and that's somewhat reassuring.

She wants to know how long she has to stay. She explains that she met the doctor today and that he said she looked really well and all her tests were fine, and that it was up to me to get her home. We talk around this one for a little while, and my father injects that we should wait and see what the doctor has to say, and that my mother being in the hospital is actually good for her, since it gives her a much-needed period of rest.

As I drive my father home, I ask him if he's really comfortable with the potential of my mother coming home tomorrow. Can he cope? Will she cope? Will those who help them cope? I explain that I'm not just tired, but I need to do my work, and work on this book, and that while I love them dearly, I can't stop my world all the time to help, as selfish as that may seem to him. He understands and says that if the medications are right, it all should work out for the best. For how long, I ask; and he responds that the next critical stage will be another traumatic event that my mother will see as a threat to any one of us, but especially to herself. He's very logical in his thinking, and I respect his mind.

So we part, and I tell him I'll either be reporting after seeing the doctor, or be bringing my mother home. He says he hopes I'll be bringing her home now that he's rested and ready. He smiles and tells me that this part of his life sure isn't what he expected it to be.

July 31, 2001

This morning I get to the hospital early and wait for the resident psychiatric doctor at the nursing station. I sit around for a while, and then look into my mother's room. She's sitting on the bed, sorting through some clothes. My strategy had been to avoid my mother and see the doctor, because I was frankly afraid of what I'd find or how things would go with her. But she looks up about the same time as I'm looking in, and she smiles and calls for me. I go in and kiss her, and she's so happy for the moment. Then she tells me that even though she's totally fine, she was told she couldn't go home today. I say that as far as I know, she maybe can go home today, but that I'm waiting and watching for the doctor to arrive, and I don't want to miss him.

My mother and I have this disjointed conversation that covers how bad the nurses are to how badly she slept to how good the food is to how well she slept to how some spies are being kept down the hall to how nice the nurses are, all in one long outpouring. But she is much calmer, and her eyes are clearer and more focused.

After a few minutes, I tell her that I should go back in the hall to wait for the doctor, and she agrees, and that's what I do.

The doctor arrives in a flurry of energy and kindly intensity. After we shake hands he tells me to follow him to someone's office way down the hall. My mother sees this and calls out to me, to tell me to help her get home, and I assure her that's utmost on my agenda.

In the office we meet with a really gentle and caring nurse and a social worker. We spend 45 minutes talking about my mother's condition, what safeguards she needs, how we need to deal with her condition, and what medications she will require. I learn that after all the many tests these past many months, and through a process of elimination, they have diagnosed my mother with Alzheimer's. She's at about mid-point, which is bad, I know, from reading the material Michael has given me and from the conversations he and I have had. In fact, the doctor tells me, most people in the same condition are institutionalized, but because my parents have care in the home and because my mother could respond to medications, remaining at home is a viable option.

Then I collect my mother so she can talk with him for a few minutes as he explains the medications he's assigned for her. I want him to do that to avoid her suggesting again that medicines are sent to her without explanation. The doctor also asks my mother how she is doing, and she assures him she feels fine and that she appreciates the help she's been given, and how she's done so well in demonstrating her mental agility through all the tests she's taken. It's a sad moment for me. Almost as an afterthought — but a good one — the doctor suggests that he give my mother an overnight pass and that we come back tomorrow for a short meeting to see how my mother's doing before she's discharged. We all agree.

Back in her room, we pack her things and wait for the nurse to bring the medications my mother needs to take until her return visit. My mother is suspicious, wondering if they will really let her leave now or if they are going to keep her again when we come back tomorrow? I assure her that everything will be just fine.

With overnight bag in hand and pill packets in my pocket, we leave the wing, but only after a long battle with the armed door, because the staff person presses the wrong button and the door won't open, which reinforces my mother's impression that she's been confined in a jail of some kind. And we head home. Along the way, we stop at a convenience store and I get a few cans of her favourite soft drink. My motive is to use my cell phone while I'm in the store to call my father and alert him about my mother's condition and what that requires of all of us.

When we arrive at my parents' house, my father is at the front door, all smiles, standing wobbly, but proud and happy. My mother works her way up the front porch steps, across the porch, and they hug and kiss. Another heart-melting moment for me, as surely it is for them.

For the next hour, we talk about my mother's experiences in the hospital, which she still thinks was a prison of some kind with spies, the too-cold air conditioning, the lack of help, the tests, and on and on. My mother says things that surprise and stun me, but I think I've learned to accept her world without challenge and debate. It's not easy, or realistic, or practical, but very necessary. As Michael and the psychiatric doctor both have said to me, it's important not to agitate a demented person, because that only serves as a trigger to another, more intense irrational reaction.

On my drive home, I think about how we baby boomers all over are facing the same kind of crisis. We're worrying about our children and we're needing to care for our parents. Some call it the sandwich generation. Whatever you call it, the fact is that we're stuck carrying a lot of baggage, a lot of worry, and a whole lot of responsibility. And guess what? It's not fun.

But then again, maybe it's not a crisis at all. Maybe it's just one more rock to roll up the hill as Sisyphus did in Greek mythology: a test of ourselves and our patience and endurance and commitment and the depth of our love for family. And if we're to pass that test, we've got to be a bit selfish. We've got to recognize that we won't be able to help our aging parents or our children if we don't take time out for ourselves. Easier said than done, yes, but critically important. As I talk and work with doctors and nurses and caregivers who are much more experienced and wiser than I am, they have one clear and consistent message: I'm the one who's delivering for them, and if I can't, it won't happen.

So what does that mean?

It means, quite simply, that if I drop the ball, it's game over for all of us, because I'll be of no use to anyone, and my parents won't get the level and range of help they need and deserve. And I will certainly drop the ball if I get too stressed out or worse, sick. Michael has talked a lot about the need to bear this in mind and to deal with it.

As I think about this, it seems to me that for those of us who, by design or default, end up as primary care givers to our parents there are three serious challenges we all face: managing the physical demands of time and stress; managing the mental drain of focusing so hard on their needs; and managing the frustration and guilt we feel as matters worsen.

To face the physical demands we have to arrange our priorities in such a way that we don't compromise the other parts of our lives. From my own experience in the past half-year especially, it's obvious that if we take on the task of helping our parents, the demands for time and attention will grow rapidly. In order to not jeopardize our other family commitments and our vocational expectations, we have to create some level of balance and set priorities. For example, I've talked to all three of my children and explained that right now I'm in a very difficult and demanding time with their grandparents, and so for a while at least, they need to understand that, I'll have less time for them. I have explained that this doesn't reflect a lack of love for them, but that it's a balancing act I hope they understand. I think they do.

On the work side, it's a matter of ensuring "the job" gets done. In my case, I'm fortunate that we have our own business and can juggle client work between Gail and me. It's also fortunate that as I'm deep into this especially trying time, we're not that busy – although that's a double-edged sword, because not being very busy also means not generating an income level we need. Others I know who are engulfed in parental caregiving and who work tell me that managing their work life has become very difficult as they need to ask for more and more time off — with consequences.

And there's one more element to the physical demands of time and stress: not losing play and rest time. We all need to play and rest. Everyone needs need to set aside some time each week to just go and do what it is they like best to do. To stop all playtime is to become vulnerable to fatigue, burn out, and illness.

Managing the mental drain of focusing so hard on our parents' needs is the second challenge. And that drain is real, even if we don't notice it. It's an unwelcome but constant companion. It eats at us, and affects our ability for sound judgment and expected behaviour. A tired, cluttered brain isn't one that's going to make logical, sound decisions. It is, one, though, that'll lead us into trouble faster than almost anything else we do.

For example, I know that I'm not as tolerant right now as I should be — with almost anyone. That bothers me, and I tell myself that I've got to watch it, but it's hard. I find I'm talking too much to too many people about what I'm experiencing. On one hand, it's probably therapeutic for me; on the other hand, I can imagine that in some cases I'm wearing out my welcome. People have their own problems and challenges to face, and clients have their own needs. So by dousing them with a stream of my personal woe, I'm not doing them any favours.

The key, it seems to me, is to understand and acknowledge the mental drain that comes with more involved caregiving, especially when a parent is suffering from physical or emotional problems. When the mental drain level soars, it's critical to take a break somehow, in some way – perhaps a quiet day, a short trip, or some kind of change to give the head and heart a break from the tension and pressure.

The third challenge — managing the frustration and guilt we feel as matters worsen — is a tough one. Feeling frustration and guilt is a natural part of caring for and loving our parents. But when either or both is physically or mentally ill, there's only so much we can do, and it's important to recognize and come to terms with that fact. While we can be supportive; while we can spend a lot of time and energy to help them, we can't turn back the clock and we can't fix the unfixable. We can be responsive and responsible, but we can't blame ourselves for what isn't our doing.

I know I'm battling frustration and guilt right now. I'm busy second-guessing what I should have done in the past couple of years, or what else I could be doing right now. But when I look at it dispassionately, there really isn't much. I give, on all levels, as much as I can, and I have to accept that there's no more I can give, short of giving up my life and focusing totally on theirs. And that's not what a parent-child relationship is all about. Rather, I keep reminding myself, that relationship is supposed to be about our parents helping rear and nurture us to a point where we're launched into our own world, to seek our own course.

That's why I, and all of us who strive to help our parents as best we can, must acknowledge that we can and will do all we can, but not suffer guilt trips. I'm learning this the hard way because my mother is trying to induce guilt right now. Demented or not, Alzheimer's or not, she's really working me over. For a long time, I didn't understand or recognize that. Now I do. That doesn't mean I love her any less; it only means I'm finally getting smarter and learning how to deal with it better.

As I near my destination, I conclude that the three challenges we face are real and threats to all of us. I've learned so much, the hard way the past few months. I know I've got to manage as best I can, and with the help of Gail and my children and our ever-expanding number of medical and social worker specialists, I will. But I do have to be "selfish" to the extent that I manage my priorities and give myself permission to look after me.

It's as simple and complex as that.

August 1, 2001

Today is my mother's birthday. She's 87.

This morning, Gail and I drive into the city; she, for appointments, and me, to take my mother to her noon appointment with the psychiatric doctor. I arrive a few minutes early to pick her up and find her tense and apprehensive. I assure her all will be right, and she snaps back that this is her birthday. My father tells me he's tired, and my mother complains that no one's called to wish her a happy birthday. I remind her that their friends know not to call before early afternoon, but this doesn't wash with her. She's clearly miffed that her birthday isn't being celebrated as she thinks it should.

We pack up my mother and her walker and I take her back to the hospital, arrive at the geriatric psychiatry wing right on time. On the way I had to listen to my mother tell me how I was late to pick her up, and how Gail says I'm always late for everything, and how it seems I can't manage my time very well, and more. After waiting awhile, the doctor arrives again in a breeze of energy, does a few things, and again asks me to come to the same office to talk about how my mother coped over the past 24 hours. I tell him I'm not sure, since I wasn't there, and I call my father to ask. He tells me in Hungarian, and I tell the doctor in English, that she was pretty tired and calm, and all things considered, everything worked out rather well.

After my report, he asks me to get my mother, which I do. He then asks her how she felt, and a lot of other questions that, as I listen, makes it clear he's probing to determine how mentally lucid she is. He explains again to her what medication to take, and gives her a list and a prescription for one new pill (to help her relax more and sleep better). He says he's arranged for a nurse to see my mother twice a week, and that he wants me to make an appointment for her to see a geriatric psychiatrist next week. Finally, he says he's signing a discharge order, and that my mother is free to go.

My mother is reasonably calm through the meeting, saying that she understands everything and is delighted to do everything. We all smile a lot and shake hands and my mother and I head back down the long hall to the security door. And as we walk down the hall, she pushing her walker and me walking next to her, she tells me again how all that's happened has been a set-up — a conspiracy — organized to do something I don't quite understand.

Once I get her back into the car, we stop at the pharmacy to drop off the prescription, and I tell her we'll have a birthday lunch. She says that would be nice and that she'd like a bowl of hot soup, but she doesn't want to go anywhere that anyone will recognize her because she can't handle the shame. I ignore this and take her to a nice suburban mall restaurant she knows. We study the menu, and my mother says she doesn't want any soup. We study the menu some more, and she says she doesn't want any kind of chicken dish, of which there are a lot. I suggest a spinach salad, and she agrees. We order and talk and it's nice and comfortable. I tell her stories about our friends, and she asks a lot of questions. Lunch arrives, and my mother digs in and eats like she hadn't seen food for a long time. Bits and pieces stick to her chin and some falls in her lap, but I say nothing.

We have a very nice time, and I'm thankful and pleased. Then, I lead her to a bench in one of the mall hallways and ask her to wait while I charge off to buy a few grocery items they need. When I get back, laden with bags, she's agitated. She needs toothpaste, she tells me — toothpaste she's asked me to get but I haven't. So I rush off to do that. When I get back, she tells me that she's tired and wants to go home because my father must surely be missing her and needing her attention. After all, my mother tells me, he's so fragile and wonderful, but she does wish he'd stop behaving so badly.

It's very hot out. We load into the car, crank up the air conditioning, and set off. We stop to pick up her new prescription, and then drive to my parents' house. When we get inside, all hell breaks loose. She's suddenly again very agitated and abusive. Everything is wrong. No one cares about her. It's her birthday and no one's called. She's ashamed to talk to anyone because she's been in a place that's locked up and her friends all know that. Where is the surprise party I said I'd arranged? And so on it goes. Then she tries on her birthday present — a new sweat suit—and it doesn't fit right, and that sets her off some more. My mother tells me with quite some intensity that she's got a lot of clothes, but none fits right, and all are old and worn. She sternly scolds their helper for holding her arm as she walks, telling her that she'll call for help when she needs it.

My father looks wan again. Sitting in the living room, he tells me how tired he is, and that he's taken some aspirin because he can feel pressure on his heart.

I just want out of there. It gets worse when my mother asks why I'm holding a container of her pills. I tell her it's one that's been replaced by what we just picked up, and we should throw it away, but she wants it to study and hold it as "evidence." I make the serious mistake of pulling it out of her hands and tossing it into the wastepaper basket This leads to a major confrontation with her saying she doesn't need her pills anyway, how her diabetes has been cured, and that no one is calling to wish her a happy birthday.

I backtrack, but it's not enough, and so I improvise as best I can. But the damage is done, and I did it, and so I tell her I'm going downtown to pick up Gail and her other birthday surprises, and we'll be back.

Two hours later my father answers the door, looking even paler than earlier in the day. He says my mother is in her bedroom. Gail and I go to see her and Gail wishes my mother a happy birthday. My mother says she's tired and wants to rest, and tells us to go away. Gail shows her the flower arrangement she brought and the cake with my mother's name inscribed. My mother wants to know why Gail didn't call her the past week. And so we go again in a futile circle of senseless and unsatisfying conversation.

Gail tells my mother she'll put the flowers in a vase, and she leaves the room while I sit by her and talk nicely about our day. My mother, though, is focused on my father — how he's being so mean to her while she's being so forgiving. We talk about this for a new minutes, and my mother says that what she needs is to hear my father say is that he loves her and that he's sorry about what he's done. Of course, he's said this a number of times over the past days, but she needs to hear it again, so I go to my father who's sitting in the living room and explain he's got to do it again. He's tired and wants to rest, but he props himself up, shuffles down the hall to her bedroom, and says it all one more time. I ask her to stand and and for them to hug and kiss, which they do. And then my mother starts again about how my father refuses to confess his bad behaviour. As I look at him, I feel a pang in my heart because I can see the hurt and the weariness on his face.

We all head back to the living room where Gail's sitting. For the next half hour, we try to make pleasant conversation about nothing in particular and admire the flower arrangement. My mother keeps delving into the most recent black hole in her mind, but she seems to be more subdued. Finally, Gail and I hug and kiss my mother and father and leave.

In the car, I call a couple of my parents' friends who understand my mother's condition. I remind them it's her birthday and ask them to call her.

And that's the way the day closes.

Tonight, as I write this, I dread the thought of the phone ringing. I don't want to hear any news. I'm tired. I'm dejected. I'm worried. I'm lost. I don't know what comes next, but whatever it is, I fear it.

On that note that I'm going to head off to sleep, convinced that tomorrow another chapter will unfold in the drama of our lives — a chapter that, if we're all fortunate, will be calmer, but who knows for sure?

September 11, 2001: A postscript

Today I took my mother to the geriatric psychiatrist who's now seeing her for the second time since I brought her home from the hospital six weeks ago. They have a wonderful visit. My mother seems at ease and sharp as a tack.

My mother talks about her memory — how she'd like to improve her ability to remember especially near-term events and issues. The doctor then asks if she'd mind taking the same test she's taken four times in the past two years that measures her cognitive abilities. My mother agrees.

The results genuinely surprise the doctor. Two years ago, on a scale that tops at 30 points, she scored about 24. The next time she scored 22, the third time she slipped to 18, and the fourth test some six months later, she was at a dangerous 14. The lower the number, the greater the short-term memory loss, and at 14, she was in serious trouble of having little retention and much confusion. And today, her score is 25 — an amazing turnaround.

In fact, the doctor tells my mother that there's no need for him to see her for two months now, because he feels she's so much better, and that her mind seems so much sharper. This is good news all around.

On the drive home, I tell my mother how proud I am of her and her progress. I explain that all the trauma of the past months is regrettable: having to take her to the hospital, having her tested, and living through all the personal emotional turmoil we all experienced. She tells me that she understands, and that she knows she's for the moment better, both physically and emotionally.

I have dinner with my parents and go for a short walk with my father, who next weeks marks his 96th birthday. And then I head home with the fervent hope that we've stabilized and that, God willing, things can be calm and all right for a time.

Yet there's always the nagging reality that both my mother and father are old and at risk, and we just don't know what tomorrow will bring.

The lessons learned

Friend, colleague, and co-author with me of another recent book, Dr. Harvey Silver always talks about the difference between tender loving care and tough loving care. An organizational psychologist, Harvey likes to explain that tender loving care is easy: we just give what's wanted, do what's expected, and keep opting out of the difficult decisions that make us all accountable and "leaders" in the truest sense. On the other hand, tough loving care demands hard decisions that take us out of our zones of comfort. Tough loving care means while we respect a person, we don't accept problem behaviours and attitudes.

When I apply those concepts to my own experience with my parents the past few months — and in particular to my mother's problems — I think the biggest, most valuable lesson I learned is that we must abide by our parents' wishes, but only so long as they don't harm themselves or each other or anyone else. There comes a critical point in time when we have to take control and do the undoable: when we have to bite the bullet and make decisions that hurt, but in fact, that will help. Had I not taken the painful steps of having my mother hospitalized against her wishes, we may well have had a family crisis that could have cost us more emotionally than we could have managed.

I also have learned that tolerance is golden. In the case of my mother, I needed to accept her concerns and fears. I didn't do that too well, and as a result I probably caused more mutual pain than was needed. But I don't think I understood that as well two months ago as I do today.

It's a delicate balancing act to exercise tough loving care. It's knowing when to intervene and where to draw the line. Common sense should've told me that, but in retrospect, there just wasn't too much common sense evident when the emotions of the moment tended to overwhelm good reasoning.

Another lesson I learned is the need to better understand what the doctors are and aren't saying. They're trying to do the best they can, and I was touched by their genuine concern and eagerness to find the best possible ways to help my mother. But because they have their own pressures, and because many well-intentioned doctors can't seem to explain things in a patient, clear way, too often we don't understand what we hear. I learned to keep asking, to seek further clarification, to, as they say, "drill down." I think I became somewhat of a pest with my persistent questioning, yet it was only because I kept asking questions that I got a much better picture of what we were facing.

Finally, I learned to slow down with my parents and to try to talk more slowly and more clearly. The more intense I'd become, the more agitated they'd become, and we'd end up in confrontational situations. While what I was saying at any time to my parents was clear to me, I was operating in my paradigm, not theirs, which I find frustrating, but I need to understand. So the more calmly I speak, the more receptive they are. It's such a simple lesson, but one that I've learned the hard way.

Personal Parenting Planner

Introduction

Inevitably, there will come a time when you will need to act promptly to help your parents in some type of emergency or a family crisis. When that time comes, you'll need to know how to access people and documents to best support your parents' needs at that moment. If you have to start searching for—or guessing about—where to find the information that's needed, you'll lose valuable time and only fuel your own level of anxiety and tension.

That's why we've included this Personal Parenting Planner. At first glance, filling in all the blanks in this extensive document may seem daunting. Or, for some, it may appear to be an unneeded or even frivolous, time-consuming task. But we would like to assure you that this Personal Parenting Planner will be an invaluable tool and resource for you at some point, in some way.

Consider all the corporations, hospitals, government departments, and most other organizations that have complex, comprehensive crisis management plans. The plans that are good all have a lot of lists—where to find people, important information about the organization, needed resources, and more. Those plans and lists exist because experience has shown that when there is any emergency situation or a full-blown crisis, it's critical to be able to find the accurate information needed to make decisions – and to find it quickly. Time becomes an essential factor, and in times of crisis, most of us won't know or remember half of what we need to have in hand.

There are two parts to the Personal Parenting Planner. Part 1 is an inventory—a fact-gathering mission to collect useful information and to assess family capabilities and commitment. Some of the considerations you'll be asked to tackle may be uncomfortable; however, now is the time to address them. Part 2 is an action plan of what you will do now and later—for your parents, and for yourself.

We've tried to make the Personal Parenting Planner as comprehensive and broad-based as possible. But remember: the Planner will be only helpful and relevant if it's updated as information changes. Don't just file it in your desk once you've completed it. Try to remember to make changes to it as they occur, and make a note on your calendar to review it every few months.

PERSONAL PARENTING PLANNER: PART 1
Taking Inventory

Last updated on: _____

Section 1: My Parents' Advisers and Friends
(In this section, list full names, addresses, telephone and fax numbers, and e-mail addresses of those people who help or advise your parents. If you don't have the information, now is the time to collect it!)

Their family physician:

_____

_____

_____

Health-related specialists they see:

_____

_____

_____

Their lawyer:

_____

_____

_____

Their accountant:

_____

_____

_____

Their bank:

_____

_____

_____

Types of accounts and account numbers:

_____

_____

_____

Safety deposit boxes *(location and number)*:

_____

_____

_____

Their sources of current income (include investment income and all pension income):

_____

_____

_____

Location of up-to-date wills:

_____

_____

_____

Location of living wills:

_____

_____

_____

Location of signed power of attorney documents:

_____

_____

_____

Their closest relatives:

_____

_____

_____

Their closest friends:

_____

_____

_____

Their immediate neighbours:

_____

_____

_____

They have made funeral arrangements through:

_____

_____

_____

They have made burial decisions, which are kept:

_____

_____

_____

Location of important family documents:

_____

_____

_____

Section 2: Profile of My Parents

(This section is an inventory of the state of your parents' health, mind-set, and observed behaviour right now. This can be a difficult section to complete. You must be as objective and honest as possible and make the best possible assumptions in some cases. The end result is a profile of each of your parents that will help you better assess their current condition and allow you to better anticipate their personal mental and physical health needs in the immediate future.)

Father

My father is ———————————years old.

His health right now is:
- ❏ good
- ❏ stable
- ❏ questionable
- ❏ eroding
- ❏ not good
- ❏ poor

His main health problems are:

_____

_____

_____

To the best of my knowledge, his doctor thinks that my father is:
- ❏ doing well for his age
- ❏ has some minor problems
- ❏ has at least one major problem
- ❏ has very serious problems

Mentally, my father is:
- ❏ sound

❑ gets confused now and then
❑ gets confused often
❑ fragile

Physically, my father's ability to move is:
❑ independent and mobile
❑ relatively stable
❑ stable but at times unsure
❑ safer with a cane
❑ safer with a walker
❑ restricted to the use of a walker
❑ very limited

If he's taking medication on a regular basis, he:
❑ is consistent and reliable
❑ sometimes forgets
❑ often forgets
❑ must be given prepackaged doses
❑ must be administered medications

Socially, my father is:
❑ active
❑ moderately active
❑ a bit passive
❑ passive
❑ reclusive

With my mother, he is:
❑ supportive
❑ fairly supportive
❑ moderately supportive
❑ not very supportive
❑ passive
❑ unsupportive
❑ hostile

With my spouse, he is:

- ❏ very comfortable
- ❏ somewhat comfortable
- ❏ not very comfortable
- ❏ somewhat uncomfortable
- ❏ very uncomfortable
- ❏ hostile

With my children, he is:

- ❏ kind and caring
- ❏ very involved
- ❏ somewhat involved
- ❏ mostly uninvolved
- ❏ totally uninvolved

With other immediate family, he is:

- ❏ very comfortable
- ❏ somewhat comfortable
- ❏ not very comfortable
- ❏ somewhat uncomfortable
- ❏ very uncomfortable
- ❏ hostile

My family would likely characterize my father as:

- ❏ nice to be with most all of the time
- ❏ nice to be with for shorter periods of time
- ❏ tolerable to be with from time to time
- ❏ not very nice to be with any time

Why?

_____

_____

_____

Usually in appearance, he is:
- ❑ well groomed
- ❑ not too well groomed
- ❑ sloppy
- ❑ dishevelled

He enjoys:
- ❑ hobbies that keep him occupied, which are:

_____

_____

_____

- ❑ some hobbies that interest him, which are:

_____

_____

_____

- ❑ a hobby that engages him periodically, which is:

_____

- ❑ no hobbies

He has:
- ❑ a number of friends he meets/talks with on a regular basis
- ❑ a few friends he meets/talks with on a regular basis
- ❑ one friend he meets/talks with on a regular basis
- ❑ a few friends he meets/talks with only infrequently
- ❑ no friends he meets/talks with on a regular basis

He:
- ❑ gets out frequently to do things
- ❑ gets out from time to time to do things
- ❑ doesn't get out much

❑ rarely gets out of the house
❑ doesn't go out at all

He:

❑ drives a car all the time
❑ drives a car at least once a week
❑ drives a car once in a while
❑ doesn't drive

When he drives, he:

❑ drives safely
❑ occasionally loses his way
❑ often loses his way
❑ drives unsafely

He:

❑ has a will that is current
❑ has a will that was written or updated within the past five years
❑ has a will that was written a number of years ago and has not been changed
❑ does not have a will

He:

❑ has given me power of attorney
❑ has not given me power of attorney
❑ has given power of attorney to _____

Overall, I think my father right now is:

in a physical condition that can be best summarized as

_____

_____

_____

in an emotional condition that can best be summarized as

_____

_____

_____

and so the most important thing I have to watch for is

_____

_____

_____

Mother

My mother is _____years old.

Her health right now is:
- ❏ good
- ❏ stable
- ❏ questionable
- ❏ eroding
- ❏ not good
- ❏ poor

Her main health problems are:

_____

_____

_____

To the best of my knowledge, her doctor thinks that my mother is:
- ❏ doing well for her age
- ❏ has some minor problems
- ❏ has at least one major problem
- ❏ has very serious problems

Mentally, my mother is:
- ❏ sound
- ❏ gets confused now and then
- ❏ gets confused often
- ❏ fragile

Physically, my mother's ability to move is:
- ❏ independent and mobile
- ❏ relatively stable
- ❏ stable but at times unsure
- ❏ safer with a cane
- ❏ safer with a walker

❏ restricted to the use of a walker
❏ very limited

If she's taking medication on a regular basis, she:

❏ is consistent and reliable
❏ sometimes forgets
❏ often forgets
❏ must be given prepackaged doses
❏ must be administered medications

Socially, my mother is:

❏ active
❏ moderately active
❏ a bit passive
❏ passive
❏ reclusive

With my father, she is:

❏ supportive
❏ fairly supportive
❏ moderately supportive
❏ not very supportive
❏ passive
❏ unsupportive
❏ hostile

With my spouse, she is:

❏ very comfortable
❏ somewhat comfortable
❏ not very comfortable
❏ somewhat uncomfortable
❏ very uncomfortable
❏ hostile

With my children, she is:

❏ kind and caring

❑ very involved
❑ somewhat involved
❑ mostly uninvolved
❑ totally uninvolved

With other immediate family, she is:
❑ very comfortable
❑ somewhat comfortable
❑ not very comfortable
❑ somewhat uncomfortable
❑ very uncomfortable
❑ hostile

My family would likely characterize my mother as:
❑ nice to be with most all of the time
❑ nice to be with for shorter periods of time
❑ tolerable to be with from time to time
❑ not very nice to be with any time

Why?

_____

_____

_____

Usually in appearance, she is:
❑ well groomed
❑ not too well groomed
❑ sloppy
❑ dishevelled

She enjoys:
❑ hobbies that keep her occupied, which are:

_____

_____

_____

❏ some hobbies that interest her, which are:

_____

_____

_____

❏ a hobby that engages her periodically, which is:

_____

❏ no hobbies

She has:

❏ a number of friends she meets/talks with on a regular basis
❏ a few friends she meets/talks with on a regular basis
❏ one friend she meets/talks with on a regular basis
❏ a few friends she meets/talks with only infrequently
❏ no friends she meets/talks with on a regular basis

She:

❏ gets out frequently to do things
❏ gets out from time to time to do things
❏ doesn't get out much
❏ rarely gets out of the house
❏ doesn't go out at all

She:

❏ drives a car all the time
❏ drives a car at least once a week
❏ drives a car once in a while
❏ doesn't drive

When she drives, she:

❏ drives safely
❏ occasionally loses her way
❏ often loses her way several times
❏ drives unsafely

She:

❑ has a will that is current

❑ has a will that was written or updated within the past five years

❑ has a will that was written a number of years ago and has not been changed

❑ does not have a will

She:

❑ has given me power of attorney

❑ has not given me power of attorney

❑ has given power of attorney to ⎯⎯⎯⎯⎯⎯⎯⎯⎯⎯⎯⎯

Overall, I think my mother right now is:

in a physical condition that can be best summarized as

⎯⎯⎯⎯⎯⎯⎯⎯⎯⎯⎯⎯⎯⎯⎯⎯⎯⎯⎯⎯⎯⎯⎯⎯⎯⎯⎯⎯⎯⎯⎯

⎯⎯⎯⎯⎯⎯⎯⎯⎯⎯⎯⎯⎯⎯⎯⎯⎯⎯⎯⎯⎯⎯⎯⎯⎯⎯⎯⎯⎯⎯⎯

⎯⎯⎯⎯⎯⎯⎯⎯⎯⎯⎯⎯⎯⎯⎯⎯⎯⎯⎯⎯⎯⎯⎯⎯⎯⎯⎯⎯⎯⎯⎯

in an emotional condition that can best be summarized as

⎯⎯⎯⎯⎯⎯⎯⎯⎯⎯⎯⎯⎯⎯⎯⎯⎯⎯⎯⎯⎯⎯⎯⎯⎯⎯⎯⎯⎯⎯⎯

⎯⎯⎯⎯⎯⎯⎯⎯⎯⎯⎯⎯⎯⎯⎯⎯⎯⎯⎯⎯⎯⎯⎯⎯⎯⎯⎯⎯⎯⎯⎯

⎯⎯⎯⎯⎯⎯⎯⎯⎯⎯⎯⎯⎯⎯⎯⎯⎯⎯⎯⎯⎯⎯⎯⎯⎯⎯⎯⎯⎯⎯⎯

and so the most important thing I have to watch for is

⎯⎯⎯⎯⎯⎯⎯⎯⎯⎯⎯⎯⎯⎯⎯⎯⎯⎯⎯⎯⎯⎯⎯⎯⎯⎯⎯⎯⎯⎯⎯

⎯⎯⎯⎯⎯⎯⎯⎯⎯⎯⎯⎯⎯⎯⎯⎯⎯⎯⎯⎯⎯⎯⎯⎯⎯⎯⎯⎯⎯⎯⎯

⎯⎯⎯⎯⎯⎯⎯⎯⎯⎯⎯⎯⎯⎯⎯⎯⎯⎯⎯⎯⎯⎯⎯⎯⎯⎯⎯⎯⎯⎯⎯

My parents together

My parents are:
- ❏ married
- ❏ separated
- ❏ divorced

As a married couple they:
- ❏ get along well all of the time
- ❏ get along well most of the time
- ❏ have a fair amount of friction between them
- ❏ argue a lot
- ❏ argue all the time
- ❏ aren't very compatible

As a separated or divorced couple:
- ❏ they have a relatively good relationship
- ❏ they have a decent, "respectful" relationship
- ❏ they have a relatively poor relationship
- ❏ they don't have a relationship at all

My parents:
- ❏ share most values and beliefs
- ❏ share some values and beliefs
- ❏ don't have as much in common as I thought
- ❏ are at odds over more than I'd assumed
- ❏ tolerate each other
- ❏ aren't close at all, when I think about it

Financially, they are:
- ❏ very secure
- ❏ somewhat secure
- ❏ not very secure
- ❏ vulnerable
- ❏ I don't know

They live in:
- ❑ a house
- ❑ an apartment
- ❑ a trailer home
- ❑ our house
- ❑ in a retirement home/community
- ❑ in a nursing home
- ❑ someone else's house (——————————————)

They get outside help from:
- ❑ a housekeeper (e.g., cleaning and cooking)
  - ❑ once a week
  - ❑ twice a week
  - ❑ three-five times a week
  - ❑ daily for several hours
  - ❑ other
- ❑ a homemaker (e.g., housekeeper duties plus care services such as dressing, bathing, etc.)
  - ❑ once a week
  - ❑ twice a week
  - ❑ other three-five times a week
  - ❑ daily for several hours
- ❑ full-time in-home support
- ❑ live-in support

In our family, the person they like the most is:

_____

In our family the person my father most trusts is:

_____

In our family, the person my mother most trusts is:

_____

Based on my analysis, it seems that my father's relationship with my mother can be described as being:

_____

_____

_____

Based on my analysis, it seems that my mother's relationship with my father can be described as being:

_____

_____

_____

Finally, based on my analysis, I think that the most important factors I have to consider, act on, or watch for are:

_____

_____

_____

Section 3: My Parents' Health Care Plans and Income Sources

(In this section, record the very important data about your parents' health coverage, life insurance particulars, and income sources. In case of illness or death, you'll need these to notify various agencies and companies about possible changes in benefit payments and reporting requirements.)

Father's social insurance number: _____

Father's health card number:_____

Mother's social insurance number:_____

Mother's health card number:_____

Pension plan details:

_____

_____

_____

CPP (Canadian Pension Plan) details:

_____

_____

_____

Annuity plans:

_____

_____

_____

Supplemental old age income:

_____

_____

_____

Optional health care coverage plans:

_____

_____

_____

Life insurance policies:

_____

_____

_____

Section 4: Me and My Family

(This section is an inventory of how prepared you and your siblings are. Because it's important to plan in advance, you're being asked to consider what challenges you may face, how you might help your parents, and how—if you've got a spouse or siblings—you'll define in advance how you will co-operate to share responsibilities. Take time to think through your answers carefully. Keep in mind that defining clear goals and roles is just as vital in our personal lives as it is in business.)

Me and My Spouse/Partner

I'm _____ years old.

I'm:

- ❑ living alone
- ❑ divorced and living alone
- ❑ married
- ❑ living common-law
- ❑ in transition

My spouse/partner supports me in understanding my parents' needs and is willing to help:

- ❑ yes
- ❑ no
- ❑ not sure

If no, why not?

_____

_____

_____

If not sure, why not?

_____

_____

_____

What I need to do to enlist his/her support and help:

_____

_____

_____

My spouse/partner has his/her own parents to help, and so, we must:
- ❑ define how we'll work together to provide care for both sets of parents
- ❑ define how much time we will allocate to each set of parents
- ❑ determine how we'll ensure we have time to spend with our children
- ❑ determine how we'll find time for ourselves
- ❑ agree on how to be mutually supportive in times of stress
- ❑ set aside some quiet time to talk this through and develop a mutually acceptable plan of action

My spouse/partner doesn't have his/her own parents to help, and so I can expect he/she will help me by:
- ❑ giving me moral support
- ❑ taking more time with the children to give me more time with my parents
- ❑ spending some time each week with my parents to give me time for other obligations
- ❑ assuming some activities (e.g., banking, bill paying, etc.) to free up more of my time

My spouse/partner has his/her own children to help, and so we must:
- ❑ agree on how to manage all our relationships
- ❑ agree on how I can help with the children, and to what extent
- ❑ agree on how he/she can help with my parents, and to what extent
- ❑ ensure the children understand the new challenges we face

My Siblings

I have the following siblings:

❑ a brother who lives in _____ and
when it comes to caring about our parent(s), feels that _____
_____

❑ another brother who lives in _____
and when it comes to caring about our parent(s), feels that
_____

❑ a sister who lives in _____ and
when it comes to caring about our parent(s), feels that _____
_____

❑ another sister who lives in _____
and when it comes to caring about our parent(s), feels that
_____

(List other siblings, if you have them.)

My siblings and I are committed to caring about my parent(s):

❑ absolutely
❑ firmly
❑ somewhat
❑ not very
❑ not at all

If there is a barrier/problem about caring for my parent(s), it's that:

❑ they don't want help, even though they need it
❑ we're not on especially good terms
❑ my work leaves me too little time for anything else
❑ my home life demands a lot of time and attention
❑ financially, we don't have extra money to spend on parental support of any kind
❑ I have a medical condition that will prevent me from providing a lot of hands-on support
❑ there is a lack of willingness among my brother(s) and/or sister(s) to help me
❑ other: _____

In terms of caring for my parents, that means:

_____

_____

_____

My sibling and I have talked about what that implies in terms of time, energy, and resources:

    ❑ yes

    ❑ not very much

    ❑ not at all

We are clear and in agreement about what we will do with and for our parents:

    ❑ yes

    ❑ not very

    ❑ not at all

I can best help my parent(s) with the following specific activities/needs: (Rank the following as 1=easy to do; 2=can do without too much difficulty; 3=can't do very easily; 4=difficult to do; 5= impossible to do)

    ___ calling on a regular basis to talk with and check on them

    ___ visiting once a week

    ___ visiting more frequently

    ___ taking them to the bank

    ___ taking them for walks

    ___ taking them for drives

    ___ taking them to social events/movies/plays/concerts

    ___ bringing them to my house for a visit

    ___ taking them for doctors' appointments

    ___ talk with their doctors regarding their health and medications

    ___ taking prescriptions to the pharmacy/picking up prescriptions

    ___ grocery shopping for them regularly

    ___ taking them for hair appointments

    ___ doing handy work/repairs around their house

    ___ cooking for them once or twice a week

__ preparing meals in advance for them weekly

__ helping with bill paying

__ helping with financial matters

__ helping with tax returns

__ arranging home repairs

__ arranging in-home support services

__ monitoring the service quality of any support services

__ gardening and lawn care

__ shovelling snow

—— _____

—— _____

—— _____

The two things I can least help my parents with are:

_____

_____

_____

_____ , my brother, can and would best help my parent(s) with: (Rank the following as 1=easy to do; 2=can do without too much difficulty; 3=can't do very easily; 4=difficult to do; 5= impossible to do)

__ calling on a regular basis to talk with and check on them

__ visiting once a week

__ visiting more frequently

__ taking them parents to the bank

__ taking them parents for walks

__ taking them parents for drives

__ taking them to social events/movies/plays/concerts

__ bring them to his house for a visit

__ taking them for doctors' appointments

__ talk with their doctors regarding their health and medications

__ taking prescriptions to the pharmacy/picking up prescriptions

__ grocery shopping for them regularly

__ taking them for hair appointments

__ doing handy work/repairs around their house
__ cooking for them once or twice a week
__ preparing meals in advance for them weekly
__ helping with bill paying
__ helping with financial matters
__ helping with tax returns
__ arranging home repairs
__ arranging in-home support services
__ monitoring the service quality of any support services
__ gardening and lawn care
__ shovelling snow

__ _____
__ _____
__ _____

The two things my brother, _____ , can least help my parents with are:

_____

_____

_____

_____ , my brother, can and would best help my parent(s) with: (Rank the following as 1=easy to do; 2=can do without too much difficulty; 3=can't do very easily; 4=difficult to do; 5= impossible to do)

__ calling on a regular basis to talk with and check on them
__ visiting once a week
__ visiting more frequently
__ taking them to the bank
__ taking them for walks
__ taking them for drives
__ taking them to social events/movies/plays/concerts
__ bring them to his house for a visit
__ take them for doctors' appointments
__ talk with their doctors regarding their health and medications

___ taking prescriptions to the pharmacy/picking up prescriptions
___ grocery shopping for them regularly
___ taking them for hair appointments
___ doing handy work/repairs around their house
___ cooking for them once or twice a week
___ preparing meals in advance for them weekly
___ helping with bill paying
___ helping with financial matters
___ helping with tax returns
___ arranging home repairs
___ arranging in-home support services
___ monitoring the service quality of any support services
___ gardening and lawn care
___ shovelling snow

___ _____
___ _____
___ _____

The two things my brother, _____, can least help
my parent(s) with are:

_____

_____

_____

_____ , my sister, can and would best
help my parent(s) with: (Rank the following as based on 1=easy to do;
2=can do without too much difficulty; 3=can't do very easily; 4=difficult
to do; 5= impossible to do)

___ calling on a regular basis to talk with and check on them
___ visiting once a week
___ visiting more frequently
___ taking them to the bank
___ taking them for walks
___ taking them parents for drives
___ taking them to social events/movies/plays/concerts

__ bring them to her house for a visit

__ take them for doctors' appointments

__ talk with their doctors regarding their health and medications

__ taking prescriptions to the pharmacy/picking up prescriptions

__ grocery shopping for them regularly

__ taking them for hair appointments

__ doing handy work/repairs around their house

__ cooking for them once or twice a week

__ preparing meals in advance for them weekly

__ helping with bill paying

__ helping with financial matters

__ helping with tax returns

__ arranging home repairs

__ arranging in-home support services

__ monitoring the service quality of any support services

__ gardening and lawn care

__ shovelling snow

__ _____

__ _____

__ _____

The two things my sister, _____ can least help my parent(s) with are:

_____

_____

_____

_____ , my sister, can and would best help my parent(s) with: (Rank the following as 1=easy to do; 2=can do without too much difficulty; 3=can't do very easily; 4=difficult to do; 5= impossible to do)

__ calling on a regular basis to talk with and check on them

__ visiting once a week

__ visiting more frequently

__ taking them to the bank

__ taking them for walks

__ taking them for drives

__ taking them to social events/movies/plays/concerts

__ bring them to her house for a visit

__ take them for doctors' appointments

__ talk with their doctors)regarding their health and medications

__ taking prescriptions to the pharmacy/picking up prescriptions

__ grocery shopping for them regularly

__ taking them for hair appointments

__ doing handy work/repairs around their house/apartment

__ cooking for them once or twice a week

__ preparing meals in advance for them weekly

__ helping with bill paying

__ helping with financial matters

__ helping with tax returns

__ arranging home repairs

__ arranging in-home support services

__ monitoring the service quality of any support services

__ gardening and lawn care

__ shovelling snow

__ _____

__ _____

__ _____

The two things my sister, _____ can least help
my parent(s) with are:

_____

_____

_____

The major challenge for me with helping my parent(s) is:

_____

   because:

_____

The major challenge for my brother _____ with helping my parent(s) is:

_____

    because:

_____

The major challenge for my brother _____ with helping my parent(s) is:

_____

    because:

_____

The major challenge for my sister _____ with helping my parent(s) is:

_____

    because:

_____

The major challenge for my sister _____ with helping my parent(s) is:

_____

    because:

_____

Given what I've discovered through this exercise, I can conclude that in the process of helping my parent(s), we will be able to do the following with consistency and care for whatever time we're needed to support them:

_____

_____

_____

_____

_____

_____

Given what I've discovered through this exercise, I can conclude that in the process of helping my parent(s), we will *not* be able to do the following with consistency and care for whatever time we're needed to support them:

_____

_____

_____

_____

_____

As a result, we must think now about how to arrange for the following:

_____

_____

_____

_____

_____

_____

PERSONAL PARENTING PLANNER: PART 2
Action Plan

Last updated on:_____

Section 1: What I need to do or plan for right now

Given what I know at the moment, **my mother** needs in the near term:
(Rank the following as 1=highest priority; 2=important to implement
soon; 3=must consider; 4=should address; 5=will probably need within
the next 9-12 months)

___ my/our added visibility and presence

___ moral support

___ help with day-to-day living

___ a "time out" from her current environment to regain her
mental and physical strength

___ specialized medical attention

___ in-home added support

___ placement in an institution

Given what I know at the moment, **my father** needs in the near term:
(Rank the following as 1=highest priority; 2=important to implement
soon; 3=must consider; 4=should address; 5=will probably need within
the next 9-12 months)

___ my/our added visibility and presence

___ moral support

___ help with day-to-day living

___ a "time out" from his current environment to regain his
mental and physical strength

___ specialized medical attention

___ in-home added support

___ placement in an institution

If either or neither parent has an up-to-date will (within the past two years), I will:

❑ help either or both update a will

❑ arrange for a lawyer to see either or both to update a will

❑ encourage my parent(s) to update a will

If either or neither parent has an up-to-date living will (within the past two years), I will:

❑ help either or both update a living will

❑ arrange for a lawyer to see either or both to update a living will

❑ encourage my parent(s) to update a living will

If either or neither parent has an up-to-date general and financial power of attorney(within the past two years), I will:

❑ help either or both update their powers of attorney

❑ arrange for a lawyer to see either or both to update their powers of attorney

❑ encourage my parent(s) to update a their powers of attorney

❑ urge my parent(s) to arrange for such powers of attorney as soon as possible

Have we discussed any special wishes **my mother** may have regarding the kind and level of health care she expects, especially in defining how to handle the question of prolonging her life if she is in a critical condition?

❑ yes, we have and have a clear understanding

❑ we've talked about it, but there is no clear direction

❑ no, we haven't talked about it

If not, I will _____

Have we discussed any special wishes **my father** may have regarding the kind and level of health care he expects, especially in defining how to handle the question of prolonging his life if he is in a critical condition?

❑ yes, we have and have a clear understanding

❑ we've talked about it, but there is no clear direction

❑ no, we haven't talked about it

If not, I will _____

We have discussed and prepared obituary notices:

❑ yes

❑ no

if not, I will _____

We have discussed how to distribute special mementoes, heirlooms, and other personal effects:

❑ yes

❑ no

if not, I will _____

Section 2: What I probably will need to do in the near future

Based on all I now know about **my mother,** I believe that within the next two years, she will need the following (in order of priority):

1. _____

2. _____

3. _____

4. _____

Of these, I can provide the following:

1. _____

2. _____

3. _____

4. _____

Of these, I will need help with the following from other sources (see Resource Directory for support agencies):

1. _____

Source: _____

2. _____

Source: _____

3. _____

Source: _____

4. _____

Source: _____

Based on all I now know about **my father,** I believe that within the next two years, he will need the following (in order of priority):

1. _____

2. _____

3. _____

4. _____

Of these, I can provide the following:

1. _____

2. _____

3. _____

4. _____

Of these, I will need help with the following from other sources (see Resource Directory for support agencies):

1. _____

Source: _____

2. _____

Source: _____

3. _____

Source: _____

4. _____

Source: _____

If and as I assume more responsibility for caring for my parents, I going to do the following for myself to ensure that I can cope most effectively:

_____

_____

_____

_____

_____

RESOURCE DIRECTORY

ONE OF THE MOST DIFFICULT AND time consuming tasks you will face when dealing with ageing parents is to identify and find the right kind of resources that offer the information, help, and support your parents need—and that *you* need in order to help them. The hard part is knowing how to locate those resources and figuring out which ones offer what services or support mechanisms.

This Resource Directory is your guide to national and provincial/territorial contacts for advice and help. There are, in fact, an amazing number of resources across Canada.. There also are many different kinds of medical specialties available to help, and they are defined in this Resource Directory in an effort to help demystify them.

While the Resource Directory is comprehensive, it doesn't attempt to be definitive, and we have refrained from trying to identify the many local support groups that exist. For those, it's best to consult your regional health authority or local hospital, or even speak with your parents' physician or your own. However, based on our research the past number of months, we believe that this Resource Directory is one of—if not the—most thorough compilations of its kind in Canada at this moment.

We have done the best we could to ensure the contact names, telepone numbers and websites are current and accurate as of March 2002.

But as we discovered, numbers and even websites are always being changed, so we're sorry for any inconvenience should you find an error.

As the challenge of caring for elderly parents continues to mushroom, there also are a growing number of local qualified individuals who—and smaller organizations that—can provide counsel and support. These are often former social workers, nurses and others who specialize in various aspects of eldercare support. Frankly, asking around is just about the best way to find them.

And finally, because so many of us are comfortable searching the web for information and resources, a word of caution: beware of all those that freely offer advice and guidance; ensure that those sites are not only current, but qualified. That, of course, takes some time and assessment on your part: demanding, yes; yet also critical to ensure that what you embrace is correct and helpful to you and your parents.

TABLE OF CONTENTS

Finding the Information You Need

This guide contains contact information for many, and are listed both by **geographical location** and by **category** or **type of service**. Many websites will lead you to other interesting and useful organizations. If you are unable to find a particular listing for your province or territory, try referring to the same category in the Canada-wide listings. National associations or organizations will be able to direct you to their closest location.

CATEGORIES

FEDERAL/PROVINCIAL/TERRITORIAL GOVERNMENT
> Government agencies that help caregivers access relevant health care services.

LONG-TERM CARE FACILITIES
> Facilities (public and private) that provide medical care to those who need it.

GENERAL RESOURCES
> A collection of helpful services and associations to help you provide better care.

NURSING AND HOMEMAKING AGENCIES
> Visiting nurses and homemakers that provide in-home assistance.

HOME HEALTH CARE RETAILERS, HOME SAFETY, AND ENVIRONMENT
> Services and retailers that provide adaptive home equipment, alarms, renovations, and more.

FINANCIAL PLANNING/LEGAL
> Organizations that will help with financial and legal matters.

VOLUNTEER AGENCIES
> Regional agencies that match volunteers with caregivers to help provide in-home or community support.

TRANSPORTATION
> Provincial/territorial ministries and driving assessment programs.

SPECIAL NEEDS

Organizations that provide services for other medical conditions (e.g., the blind or deaf population).

CARING FOR YOURSELF

Counselling and support services (e.g., crisis lines and support groups) for the caregiver.

PROFESSIONAL SERVICES

Professional colleges and associations that refer caregivers to health care professionals in their area (e.g., an occupational therapists or social workers).

Your Guide to
Health Professionals

When it comes to caring for your parents, you're not alone. There are many qualified health care professionals ready to help, each with their own special expertise.

Here's a quick introduction to the health professionals you may encounter in your caregiving journey.

Occupational Therapist

Occupational therapists focus on helping people be as engaged as possible in activities and occupations that are meaningful to them. This is based on the individual's abilities, needs and interests. As a person becomes more dependent, the occupational therapist will continue to work collaboratively with you and other caregivers. They'll help to develop a safe and supportive environment that encourages your parents to participate in their life as much as they are able by identifying customized solutions that could include recommendations about modifying tasks and/or environments and the use of assistive devices such as wheelchairs and bathroom equipment. The therapist may help you to identify strategies to make sure that you are looking after your needs as well, in your role as the caregiver.

For more information: Canadian Association of Occupational Therapists 1-800-434-2268, or the web site at www.caot.ca

Physicians

Family Physician

Family physicians provide continuing and comprehensive general medical care, health maintenance and preventive services to individuals. They are involved in co-ordinating medical care.

The family physician will know your parents' medical condition. Because of the physician's familiarity with the person, family physicians are best qualified to serve as an advocate in all health-related matters, including the appropriate use of consultants, health services, and community resources.

For more information: The College of Family Physicians of Canada 1-800-387-6197, or the web site at www.cfpc.ca

Geriatrician

In Quebec, a geriatrician is a physician specially trained in the health needs and problems of the elderly. Most geriatricians are internists or family physicians certified in geriatric medicine.

Family physicians and local hospitals are your best sources for finding the kind of geriatricians you may need.

Neurologist

A neurologist is a physician with specialized training in diagnosing, treating and managing disorders of the brain and nervous system. Neurologists treat a variety of disorders of the nervous system, including Alzheimer's disease.

A neurologist will diagnose the condition, determine the proper treatment and work with the family physician and others in managing a patient's overall health.

Psychiatrist

A psychiatrist is able to diagnose and treat behavioral and emotional challenges that result from any form of dementia which may be emerging in a parent, or which may have been present for some time. Psychiatrists are medical doctors with extra training in psychiatry and are thus able to prescribe medication for treatment.

Physiotherapist

Physiotherapists, also known as physical therapists, are health care professionals trained in the study of rehabilitation who evaluate, restore and maintain physical function.

They have a detailed understanding of how the body works and are trained to assess and improve movement and function, and relieve associated pain.

For more information: Canadian Physiotherapy Association 1-800-387-8679 or the web site at www.physiotherapy.ca

Psychologists

Psychologists specialize in treating behavioural, emotional and motivational problems. They can assess cognitive dysfunctions and recommend non-drug treatments. They also can recommend intervention programs.

Psychologists who work with clients are sometimes called Clinical Psychologists. Neuropsychologists specialize in the diagnosis of brain disorders.

For more information: Canadian Psychological Association 1-613-237-2144 or the web site at www.cpa.ca

Registered Nurses/Registered Nursing Assistants

Registered Nurses and Registered Nursing Assistants are often involved in the care and treatment of persons with any health-related need. From providing direct clinical care in the home or hospital, to providing information and counselling and helping to assess overall health needs, nursing professionals can help you to develop a comprehensive plan for care.

Nurses can help with medical and medication issues and can help you arrange for support services, such as home support, respite care and day programs. Nurses work closely with physicians and are key members of the team. A registered nursing assistant or a home health aide may also provide in-home care under the direction of a registered nurse.

For more information: Canadian Nursing Association 1-800-361-8404 or the web site at www.cna-nurses.ca

Social Workers

Social workers help individuals, families, groups and communities resolve problems that affect their well-being on an individual or collective basis. They focus on the relationships between people and their environments, helping enhance problem-solving and coping capacities.

For individuals and families coping with the challenge of ageing parents, social workers offering counselling for crisis intervention when health and safety are at risk and for loss and grief. As well, they are able to play a helpful role to caregivers to access support services.

For more information: Canadian Association of Social Workers 1-613-729-6668 or the web at www.casw-acts.ca

Speech-Language Pathologists/Audiologists

These professionals specialize in speech, language and hearing disorders.

Speech-language pathologists help individuals overcome and prevent communication problems in language, speech, voice, and fluency. Audiologists assess the extent of any hearing loss, balance and related disorders and recommend appropriate treatment.

For more information: Canadian Association of Speech Language Pathologists and Audiologists 1-800-259-8519 or the web site at www.caslpa.ca

Canada-wide

FEDERAL GOVERNMENT

Reference Canada
1-800-667-3355, or
1-800-622-6232

A central source of information on **all** federal government resources programs. Telephone lines are staffed by information officers who will direct you to federal programs, information sources and services.

Health Canada
Provides information on a broad range of health-related issues. Check the web site at www.hc-sc.gc.ca, then under the Just for You heading, click on 'Seniors', or call the Division of Aging and Seniors at -613-952-7606

GENERAL RESOURCES

Alzheimer Society of Canada
1-800-616-8816
www.alzheimer.ca

The Society offers a nation-wide network of support to individuals in groups and one-to-one and helps people find programs and services (day and respite programs, home support and help with the difficult transition to long-term care), a nation-wide Alzheimer Wandering Registry, and many educational tools and resources that are available for caregivers.

The Arthritis Society

1-800-321-1433

www:arthritis.ca

The Society provides a range of treatment and education programs from branches across Canada.

Canadian Home Care Association

613-569-1585

www.cdnhomecare.on.ca

CHCA focuses on the advancement of quality home and community-care nationally through information and knowledge sharing in order to facilitate best practices at all levels.

Canadian Mental Health Association

National office: 416-484-7750

www.cmha.ca

The CMHA focuses on combating mental health problems and emotional disorders through more than 10,000 volunteers and staff in 135 local branches across Canada.

Canadian Health Network

www.canadian-health-network.ca

CHN is a national Internet-based health information service with links to some 10,000 health-related resources.

The Heart and Stroke Foundation

National office: 613-569-4361

www.heartandstroke.ca

A federation of independent Provincial foundations and the national office, the organization has more than 250,000 volunteers dedicated to improving health by preventing and reducing disability and death from heart disease.

Canadian Red Cross Society

National office: 613-740-1900

www.redcross.ca

The Canadian Red Cross provides a number of home care services and equipment loans for eligible persons. One example is the Home Support Service: a complete program of in-home care services which provide personal care and assistance. Services vary by region; call the national office to be referred to a regional office to find what specific services are offered in your area.

Canadian Cancer Society

1-888-939-3333

www.cancer.ca

The toll-free line is a good entry point for those with questions, and to learn the telephone number of your local divisional office. Each office provides various kinds of support and services.

Canadian Diabetes Association

1-800-BANTING

www.diabetes.ca

With more than 150 branches across Canada, the Association supports research, education and advocacy for and on behalf of those with various levels ofdiabetes.

Canadian National Institute for the Blind

National office: 416-486-2500

www.cnib.ca

The CNIB is a national volunteer agency provides a range of services to those suffering from varying degrees of loss of vision, with offices across Canada. It offers numerous resources including counselling and referral, orientation and mobility training, sight enhancement, and technical aids.

Meals on Wheels

This program provides hot meals delivered to seniors in their homes. There are hundreds of Meals on Wheels programs across Canada. To find the program nearest you, please check your local phone directory or ask your care co-ordinator or family physician.

Medbroadcast Corporation

1-877-502-4400

www.medbroadcast.com

This Vancouver-based company specializes in providing online consumer health and wellness information and services

Mental Health Online

www.mentalhealth.com

Internet Mental Health is a free encyclopedia of mental health information created by a Canadian psychiatrist, Dr. Phillip Long.

Salvation Army

National office: 416-425-2111

www.salvationarmy.ca

This organization provides pastoral care visits upon request. It also operates some long term care facilities, respite care programs, and day away programs in co-operation with local health care authorities. Services vary from region to region.

Veterans' Affairs Canada

1-800-387-0919

www.vac-acc.gc.ca/general

The Veterans Independence Program provides special home care services to Canadian Veterans. Services range from transportation, home adaptations, counselling and health care to house cleaning and maintenance. There are income qualifications for specific services.

NURSING AND HOMEMAKING AGENCIES

Both non-profit and private nursing agencies provide nursing and support personnel to clients in their homes. A case manager/care co-ordinator from your regional health authority, local Community Care Access Centre or Centres Locaux de Service Communitaires will provide a needs assessment to determine if funding is available.

A variety of funded services are available including nursing, home making, respite and personal care. For example, personal support workers are often provided for people with physical disabilities, advancing dementia or Alzheimer's to help with household chores and/or personal care.

You can also purchase extra help by contacting a local nursing agency directly and arranging to pay for the services you need to supplement those paid for by the government resources. Ask your health professional for names of local agencies of contacts.

Some examples of cross-Canada agencies are:

Bayshore Health Care
1-800-461-5586
www.bayshore.ca
A private nursing agency with a full range of nursing and homemaking services.

Caregivers.Ca
National office: 416-788-CARE
www.caregivers.ca
This private firm helps families find caregivers from dozens of countries and arranges all related immigration matters.

Comcare Health Services
800-663-5775
www.comcarehealth.ca
A private nursing agency with a full range of nursing and homemaking services.

Extendicare (Canada) Inc.

Head office: 905-470-4000

www.extendicare.com

One of North America's largest operators of long-term care facilities, Extendicare has facilities across most of Canada.

ParaMed Home Health Care

1-800-465-5054

www.extendicare.com

A private nursing agency with a full range of nursing and homemaking services.

Victorian Order of Nurses (VON)

1-888-866-2273

www.von.ca

A non-profit agency. In addition to traditional nursing services, most provincial branches of the VON provide day-away programs for persons with dementia. These programs give caregivers a break while providing their clients with an opportunity to socialize and maintain their independence.

We Care Home Health Care Services

Head office: 416-922-7601

www.wecare.ca

A private agency offering franchised nursing and homemaking services across Canada.

HOME HEALTH CARE RETAILERS, HOME SAFETY, AND ENVIRONMENT

A variety of home health care products and services are available from national retailers and also from your local pharmacy. Depending on your location, many stores offer in-home assessments, equipment trials, and rental programs for short-term needs.

Your health professional should be able to refer you to local stores, or you can call and ask one of the following national retailers for the location closest to your home.

As well, there are government support programs and a Canada Post alert program that are worth exploring as the need arises.

Canada Mortgage and Housing Corporation (CMHC)

1-800-668-2642

www.cmhc.ca

CMHC's Home Adaptations for Seniors Independence (HASI)is designed to provide information and fund home adaptations related to accessibility for seniors. A maximum of $2500 is provided to qualified applicants (based on gross household income) for fixed items such as ramps, stair glides, and grab bars. It also has a Residential Rehabilitation Assistance Program for Persons with Disabilities (RRAP) with differing levels of financial assistance for homeowners and landlords who are modifying dwellings for occupancy by low-income persons with disabilities.

The programs are administered on a provincial/municipal level depending on the region. In some areas, there is supplemental funding from the province as well.

Canada Post – Letter Carrier's Alert Program

1-800-267-1177

www.canadapost.ca

Canada Post's letter carriers keep an eye on customers and report whether they detect an unusual buildup of mail or newspapers at the customers' residences. This service is free in participating communities. Contact your local postmaster or call the toll-free number and ask a customer service representative if there is a program in your area.

Canadian MedicAlert Foundation

1-800-668-1507 (English) or 1-800-668-6381 (French)

www.medicalert.ca

The Canadian MedicAlert Foundation provides service and protection to Canadians with medical needs and personal requests that should be known in the event of a medical emergency, including medical conditions, drug and food allergies, special needs and medications.

Lifecall of Canada

1-800-661-5433

www.lifecall.ca

Lifecall is an emergency response service that provides immediate attention to seniors in need. It can offer peace of mind for caregivers and family members; however seniors must remember to use the service. There is a fee.

Lifeline Systems Canada Inc.

1-800-451-0525

www.lifeline.ca

Personal response service for people living at home alone or at risk. A portable alarm button is linked by telephone line to a central call centre. There is a fee.

MEDIchair, Canada's Wellness Store

1-800-667-0087

www.medichair.com

There are MEDIchair locations from coast to coast providing a full range of medical equipment for assisted daily living.

Motion Group

1-800-267.2920

www.themotiongroup.com

More than 30 specialized providers of seating, patient room equipment and mobility products and a variety of assistive devices for persons with disabilities.

Shoppers Home Health Care

1-800-363-1020

www.shoppersdrugmart.ca

A network of specialized stores that offer a wide variety of home health care and wellness products for safety, comfort, and independence. Professionally trained staff work with you to assess your needs. Home visits are available without charge.

FINANCIAL PLANNING/LEGAL

The following organizations will refer you to trained professionals in your region who will assist you with general information you may need, and on various aspects of estate and financial planning as well as protecting your rights.

Canada Customs and Revenue Agency (formerly Revenue Canada)

1-800-267-6999

www.ccra-adrc.gc.ca

Government agency responsible for all tax matters within Canada. Maintains taxation records as well as information on Canada Pension Plan.

Canadian Association of Financial Planners

1-800-346-2237

www.cafp.org

Professionals who can provide assistance with overall financial planning. Publishes *Consumer Guide to Financial Planning and Membership Directory*.

Canadian Institute of Chartered Accountants

1-800-268-3793

www.cica.ca

The Institute will provide a listing of accounting firms by geographical information.

Certified General Accountants Association of Canada

1-800-663-1529

www.cga-canada.org

This group will refer you to the proper provincial association which will, in turn, provide a list of accountants within a local area.

Operation Phone Busters

1-888-495-8501

www.phonebusters.com

A free, national telephone service that helps fight telemarketing fraud. Offers free video information tapes and pamphlets.

VOLUNTEER AGENCIES

Tetra Society of North America
Tel: 604-688-6464
www.tetrasociety.org (under construction)

The Tetra Society matches community volunteers with people with special needs. These volunteers then create custom-designed assistive devices to help improve the individual's daily life.

SPECIAL NEEDS

The associations and foundations below offer a wealth of information and contacts on specific conditions other than dementia.

The Aphasia Institute
416-226-3636
www.aphasia.ca
The Institute helps those with a language disorder resulting from an injury to the brain—most often a stroke. Offers direct services in the greater Toronto area but can help with training and communications resources across Canada.

Canadian Association of the Deaf (CAD)
National office: 613-565-2882
www.cad.ca (under construction)
A national consumer group that provides a research and information centre, a self-help society, and a community action organization.

Canadian Continence Foundation
1-800-265-9575
www.continence-fdn.ca
The Canadian Continence Foundation offers a wealth of information on incontinence management and treatment, including books, videos, audio tapes, and newsletters. The foundation will also put you

in touch with health care professionals who have expertise with urinary incontinence.

Canadian Hard of Hearing Association

1-800-263-8068

www.chha.ca

This association provides information and brochures on improving communication skills and helping people deal with hearing loss. There is a senior's manual with helpful advice available for $4.00 per copy.

Canadian National Society of the Deaf-Blind

National contact: 905-763-6736

www.cnsdb.ca

Distributes information to help the deaf-blind and those who are caring for them.

Canadian Hospice Palliative Care Association

1-800-668-2785

Web:www.cpca.net

The association provides leadership in hospice palliative care, which is aimed at relief of suffering and improving the quality of life for those living with or dying from advanced illness or are bereaved.

Dietitians of Canada

National office tel: 416-596-0857

www.dietitians.ca

Dietitians provide tips on nutrition and eating management. The organization doesn't provide names over the phone; however, you can visit the Web site and search for a dietitian in their local area.

Dying with Dignity

1-800-495-6156

www.web.net/dwd

This organization educates caregivers on the rights of their loved ones as they near the end of life. They also provide counselling and information on living wills, advance health care directives and power of attorney.

They can refer caregivers to a local health care professional with specialized training in "end-of-life care."

Osteoporosis Society of Canada

1-800-463-6842 (English) or

1-800-977-1778 (French)

www.osteoporosis.ca

The Society assists people who have osteoporosis, and those who are at risk. Services include free publications; a bilingual, toll-free information line; educational programs; and referrals to self-help groups and community resources.

CARING FOR YOURSELF

CARP

1-800-363-9736

www.50plus.com

A national association for those 50 and older with a range of services.

The Canadian Caregiver Coalition

1-888-866-2273

www.ccc-ccan.ca

This is an alliance of individuals, groups and organizations that promotes awareness and action to address the needs of caregivers of all ages across Canada, and to influence policy.

The Caregiver Network (CNI)

National office: 416-323-1090

www.caregiver.on.ca

Based in Toronto the goal of CNI is to be a national single information source to make your life as a caregiver easier.

Caregiver Resources

www5.biostat.wustl.edu/alzheimer/submit/caregive.html

A fairly comprehensive listing of Canadian and American internet links on caregiver related topics. (Provided by the Washington University School of Medicine.)

Family Caregiver Alliance

www.caregiver.org

An American website with interesting information for family caregivers.

Resources for Caregivers

www.cp-tel.net/pamnorth

Small but useful web based resource links provided by an American hospice nurse.

Solutions – a boomer's guide to work and life balance

Publication office: 416-421-7944

www.parentcare.ca

This magazine is published six times a year and positions itself as Canada's family guide to home health care and wellness. It provides readers with a host of tips and tactics on the challenges of caring for ageing parents, as well as product and literature reviews. Solutions expects to have a special web site on line by mid summer, 2002, that will allow users access to more than 30,000 support resources that provide a wide range of eldercare services.

British Columbia

GOVERNMENT

There are a variety of non-profit and private organizations contracted through British Columbia's Regional Health Authorities that can provide home support services. They range from minimal home care to homemaking and full-time, live-in care. They also offer supervision, respite, and personal support for persons with dementia.

For general information, call the BC Ministry of Health Services at 1-800-465-4911, or visit its web site at www.healthservices.gov.bc.ca.

Office for Seniors

250-952-1238, or 1-800-465-4911

www.hlth.gov.bc.ca/seniors

Responsible for informing the public on government policies and programs for seniors.

The Information for Seniors guide is available online at www.hlth.gov.bc.ca/seniors/info. This is a comprehensive guide to programs and benefits in British Columbia.

The Ministry of Health Services also can direct you to the Regional Health Authority in your area; call the BC Ministry of Health information line at 1-800-465-4911. Or, find contacts for the five Authorities at www.healthplanning.gov.bc.ca/socsec/contacts.html

Human Resources Development Canada

For service in English: 1-800-277-9914

For service in French: 1-800-277-9915

www.bc.hrdc-drhc.gc.ca

HRDC administers two income assistance programs for seniors through its Income Security Programs (CPP & OAS).

Veterans Affairs

Services in English 604-666-7942

Services in French 604-666-2946

For information on Veteran Affairs programs contact the BC district office of Veterans Affairs Canada. Refer to GENERAL RESOURCES in the Canada-wide listings for a description of services offered.

The Canadian Seniors Policies and Programs Database

www.sppd.gc.ca

The SPPD is an Internet based database of government policies and programs for which seniors are the primary beneficiaries. It was developed and is maintained by federal, provincial and territorial governments.

LONG-TERM CARE FACILITIES

In British Columbia, long-term care is offered at extended care facilities throughout the province. Each facility has a specific number of multi-level care beds that offer varying levels of care.

The first step is to call your local regional Health Authority and request an assessment. The assessment will help determine the level of care your parents require and any other needs. Admission to a facility is based on this assessment.

To locate your local regional Health Authority, call the BC Ministry of Health information line at 1-800-465-4911 or go to www.health-planning.gov.bc.ca/socsec/contacts.html

GENERAL RESOURCES/SPECIAL NEEDS

Alzheimer Society of British Columbia

604-681-6530

1-800-667-3742

www.alzheimerbc.org

Provides educational and support programs to improve awareness and assist families and individuals coping with the disease. The society offers telephone support for families and caregivers throughout the province. Regional representatives, respite managers, and volunteers can be contacted by phone or by visiting a regional resource centre. An information package with more local material and a comprehensive facilities list can be requested at no charge.

The British Columbia Aphasia Centre

604-877-8066

Supports those with speech and language difficulties usually associated with strokes.

Arthritis Society BC & Yukon Division

604-714-5550

1-800-321-1433

www.arthritis.ca/bc

A non-profit organization devoted solely to funding and promoting arthritis research, patient care and public education.

Canadian Cancer Society BC & Yukon District Office

604-872-4400 or 1-800-663-2524

Cancer Information Line1-888-939-3333

www.bc.cancer.ca

Each divisional office provides various kinds of support and advice; call to find out what is available.

The Canadian Deafblind & Rubella Association

250- 426-2458

www.cdbra.ca

Provides intervention services to deaf-blind and rubella handicapped people throughout British Columbia.

The Canadian Diabetes Association,
604-732-133 or
1-800-665-6526
www.diabetes.ca
A national, independent, self-financing organization, works to improve the quality of life of Canadians affected by diabetes by being the leading force in research, service, advocacy and education.

Canadian Hard of Hearing Association — BC branch.
604-795-3665
www2.vpl.vancouver.bc.ca/dbs/cod/orgpgs/5/579.html
Provides information and brochures on improving communication skills and helping people deal with hearing loss

The Canadian National Institute for the Blind .
604-431-2020
www.cnib.ca/divisions/bc_yukon
A charitable, non-profit, voluntary agency that provides rehabilitation and support services to persons who are blind and visually impaired.

The Canadian Red Cross Society
250-382-2043
1-800-661-9055
Offers a variety of services to seniors.

Mental Health Information Line
604-688-3234 or
1-800-661-2121
www.cmha-bc.org
Offers information on provincial mental health programs, as well as a listing of professionals and community services

Senior Information Centre.

604-875-6381

Provides information on associations, resources, and organizations. It is for people who reside in the Lower Mainland only

Seniors Medication Information Line (BC Smile)

604-822-1330 (Vancouver) or

1-800-668-6233 (toll free in BC)

Operated by University of British Columbia licensed pharmacists, the Line assists seniors and their caregivers with drug-related questions, especially questions requiring extensive research (e.g., new medications, interactions, side effects, herbs, and vitamins).

SeniorsCan

www.crm.mb.ca/index.html

The SeniorsCan Internet Program is a highly acclaimed guide for retirees and older adults to Canadian and global information and services.

Western Institute for the Deaf and Hard of Hearing

1-888-736-7391 or

604-736-7391

An information and service resource to people who are deaf and hard of hearing and to concerned individuals and agencies.

NURSING AND HOMEMAKING AGENCIES

For nursing and homemaking agencies in your area, please refer to NURSING AND HOMEMAKING AGENCIES in the Canada-wide listings.

HOME HEALTH CARE RETAILERS, HOME SAFETY, AND ENVIRONMENT

There are a number of home health care retailers located throughout the province that can help you find the right products for your specific needs. To find a store near you, please refer to HOME HEALTH CARE RETAILERS, HOME SAFETY, AND ENVIRONMENT in the Canada-wide listings.

FINANCIAL PLANNING/LEGAL

ABC's of Fraud Program
Tel: 604-437-1940
This program gives group presentations to educate seniors about fraud. They distribute complimentary support materials and provide referrals to additional resources.

Community Legal Assistance Society
604-685-3425
Provides free legal assistance to people who are physically, mentally, or economically disadvantaged throughout BC.

Legal Services Society
604-601-6000
Non-profit organization providing legal services to people who can't afford a lawyer and legal education and legal information to the residents of BC.

Office of the Public Guardian and Trustee
604-660-4444
This office is responsible for protecting the financial rights of cognitively challenged people. They help individuals make decisions on personal care and medical treatment. The office also advises family members on guardianship and on how to obtain the legal authority to make decisions on behalf of loved ones.

VOLUNTEER AGENCIES

Senior Link

250-382-4331

This is a referral telephone help-line offering free information for residents of the Capital Health Region. Volunteers provide support as well as information and referral to all of the non-medical emergency resources available in the region. Senior Link provides personalized advice and expertise on many issues, including financial assistance, government services, housing, legal, personal support services, etc.

Seniors Resource Directory

www.seniors-internet.com/seniorsorg.html

A web-based resource directory for BC seniors.

TRANSPORTATION

In each province, the Ministry of Transportation makes the official decision on when a person must stop driving. The family physician is *legally* required to report any case in which someone's driving ability may be impaired due to the progression of age or any resulting condition. The physician must file his or her report with a Medical Review Board, which may, based on research and interviews with key health care professionals, request a driving assessment to determine driving skills. Based on test results, a decision will be made on whether the individual will be allowed to continue to drive.

If you are concerned about your parents' ability to drive, you can request an independent assessment for one or both of them. Such assessments, which are provided by private companies for a fee, will help you determine your parent's safety while on the road.

BC Ministry of Transportation and Highways, Motor Vehicles Branch

250-978-8300

The government ministry that provides driver assessments to determine competence levels.

DriveAble Testing Location
604-921-3355

Driver assessment program for persons with possible cognitive impairment. Fee for service.

CARING FOR YOURSELF

Caregivers Association of BC (CABC)
604-490-4812

CABC offers support, education, and information to unpaid family caregivers in BC. Also provides training, manuals, reports, and other educational kits to help community leaders. Publishes *BC Caregiver News*.

Community Home Support Services Association
604-739-4300

This association provides home support services and workers for caregivers of, and for people with dementia.

The Self-Help Resource Association of BC
604-733-6186

A collection of groups that focus on various physical and mentail health related issues and challenges.

The Seniors' Foundation of British Columbia
604-685-4403

www.seniorsbc.com

The Seniors' Foundation of British Columbia is committed to provide funding for projects that help seniors help themselves.

Alberta

GOVERNMENT

Access to All Provincial Government programs

You can contact any provincial government program by calling the Alberta Government "RITE" line telephone service. To use this toll-free service from anywhere in Alberta, simply dial: 310-0000 and then enter the telephone number you need, or dial zero for RITE assistance. If you do not have a touch-tone telephone, stay on the line and an operator will help you place your call.

The toll-free <u>Alberta Seniors Information Line and Seniors Service Centres</u> offer comprehensive information on programs and services for seniors in Alberta. Toll-free in Alberta: 1-800-642-3853, Edmonton area: 780-427-7876, or go the the website at www.seniors.gov.ab.ca

In Alberta, any one of the 17 <u>Regional Health Authorities</u> is a good first point of entry to the health care system. The local Health Authority in your area will conduct an assessment, and then based on the results, will direct you to the resources you need. In addition, there are a number of independent associations and organizations (such as nursing agencies) which contract work through the Health Authority. You may be able to access these private services directly and pay for any additional care you require. To locate the Health Authority in your area, call 780-310-0000, or go to www.health.gov.ab.ca/rhas/rhamap.htm for a complete listing and links.

Acute and Long-Term Care Division
780-427-5206
This division is responsible for long-term care centres which provide regular treatment services and continuing nursing care. Albertans are eligible for long-term care when they are no longer able to live independently within their communities.

Alberta Health and Wellness
780-310-0000
This department provides information on provincial health services and departments related to home care and caring for persons special needs.

Home Support Alberta
403-423-2831
Twenty offices throughout the province provide a variety of home support services. Call for contact information for your local office.

Seniors Housing Services
Edmonton: 780-427-4190
Calgary : 403-297-5399
310-0000 for toll-free service.
Facilitates the provision of adequate and affordable housing to those seniors in Alberta who need help in this area.

Human Resources Development Canada
English: 1-800-277-9914
French: 1-800-277-9915
www.ab.hrdc-drhc.gc.ca
Email: isp-psr.mail-poste@hrdc-drhc.gc.ca
HRDC administers two income assistance programs for seniors through its Income Security Programs (CPP & OAS).

Veterans Affairs

For information on Veteran Affairs programs contact the Alberta district office of Veterans Affairs Canada. Refer to GENERAL RESOURCES in the Canada-wide listings for a description of services offered. Call 403-292-4048 (Calgary) or 780-495-3762 (Edmonton) or 1-800-665-8717.

The Canadian Seniors Policies and Programs Database

www.sppd.gc.ca

The SPPD is an Internet based database of government policies and programs for which seniors are the primary beneficiaries. It was developed and is maintained by federal, provincial and territorial governments. Additional information regarding seniors organizations in Alberta is listed in the Directory of Alberta's Seniors Organizations. For a copy of the publication, contact the Alberta Seniors Information Line at 1-800-642-3853, or in Edmonton 780-427-7876.

LONG-TERM CARE FACILITIES

There are a number of facilities throughout the province which provide varying levels of care. Your local Regional Health Authority has a complete list. Your care co-ordinator will be able to direct you to the proper facility based on the level of care that your parents may need.

You also can contact the Alberta Long Term Care Association, whose members represent the public, private and voluntary sectors in the province; call 1-888-212-4581, or go to www.longtermcare.ab.ca

GENERAL RESOURCES

The Alberta Council on Aging
1-888-423-9666 or 780-423-9666 in Edmonton
www.seniorfriendly.ca
E-mail: acaging@interbaun.com
A province-wide charitable organization of groups and individuals concerned with the process of aging.

Alberta Association for Community Living

1-800-252-7556

This organization helps individuals with a developmental disability who are aging. Support services and counselling are based on need.

Alzheimer Society of Alberta

403-250-1303

1-888-233-0332

www.alzheimer.ab.ca

E-mail: provincial@alzheimer.ab.ca

The Alzheimer Society provides educational and support programs to improve awareness and to assist families and individuals coping with the disease. The resource centre is open to the public. It can provide referrals to support groups in your local area and will mail information.

The **Arthritis Society** is a non-profit organization devoted solely to funding and promoting arthritis research, patient care and public education.

403-228-2571 Toll Free 1-800-321-1433

www.arthritis.ca

E-mail: info@ab.arthritis.ca

Canadian Cancer Society Alberta NWT Division

403-228-4487

1-888-661-2261

Cancer Information Services 1-888-939-3333

www.cancer.ab.ca

E-mail: info@cancer.ab.ca

The Canadian Deafblind & Rubella Association

403-529-6454

www.cdbra.ca

Provides intervention services to deaf-blind and rubella handicapped people throughout Alberta.

The Canadian Diabetes Association

780-423-1232 or

1-800-563-0032

www.diabetes.ca

A national, independent, self-financing organization, works to improve the quality of life of Canadians affected by diabetes by being the leading force in research, service, advocacy and education.

Canadian Hard of Hearing Association — Calgary branch

403-781-6905

The association provides information and brochures on improving communication skills and helping people deal with hearing loss.

The Canadian Mental Health Association.

780-482-6576

www.cmha.ab.ca

CMHA promotes the mental health of all people and to serve mental health consumers, their families and friends.

The Canadian National Institute for the Blind

Telephone 403-488-4871

www.cnib.ca

A charitable, non-profit, voluntary agency that provides rehabilitation and support services to persons who are blind and visually impaired.

The Canadian Red Cross Society

Calgary: 403-541-6100

Edmonton: 780-423-2680

Website: www.redcross.ca

Offers a variety of services to seniors throughout the province including homecare, meals-on-wheels, equipment loan programs and a unique home partner program.

Heart and Stroke Foundation of Alberta.

403-264-5549

www.heartandstroke.ca

Provides free literature on a wide range of topics such as controlling stress, cholesterol, managing high blood pressure and smoking cessation

The Multiple Sclerosis Society of Canada

1-800-268-7582

Edmonton: 780-463-1190

www.mssociety.ca

Undertakes research into the cause and cure of multiple sclerosis and works to educate the public about the condition.

The Health Line

1-877-600-2100

www.thehealthline.com

The Alberta Consumer Health Information Society established this service as a telephone and web-based access to current health information free of charge.

NURSING AND HOMEMAKING AGENCIES

For nursing and homemaking agencies in your area, please refer to NURSING AND HOMEMAKING AGENCIES in the Canada-wide listings.

HOME HEALTH CARE RETAILERS, HOME SAFETY, AND ENVIRONMENT

There are a number of home health care retailers located throughout the province that can help you find the right products for your specific needs. To find a store near you, please refer to HOME HEALTH CARE RETAILERS, HOME SAFETY, AND ENVIRONMENT in the Canada-wide listings.

Canada Mortgage and Housing Association — Alberta Division

780-482-6576

See the Canada-wide listing under HOME HEALTH CARE RETAILERS, HOME SAFETY, AND ENVIRONMENT for services offered.

FINANCIAL PLANNING/LEGAL

ABC's of Fraud Program

403-266-6200

This program gives group presentations to educate seniors about fraud. They distribute complimentary support materials and provide referrals to additional resources.

Public Guardian and Trustee

780-427-2744

This office is responsible for protecting the financial rights of cognitively challenged people. They help individuals make decisions on personal care and medical treatment. The office also advises family members on guardianship and on how to obtain the legal authority to make decisions on behalf of loved ones.

TRANSPORTATION

In each province, the Ministry of Transportation makes the official decision on when a person must stop driving. The family physician is ethically required to report any cases in which someone's driving ability may be impaired due to the progression of age or any resulting condition. The physician must file his or her report with a Medical Review Board, which may, based on research and interviews with key health care professionals, request a driving assessment to determine driving skills. Based on test results, a decision will be made on whether the individual is allowed to drive.

If you are concerned about your parents' ability to drive, you can request an independent assessment for one or both of them. Such assessments, which are provided by private companies for a fee, will help you determine your parents' safety while on the road.

Alberta Department of Transportation and Utilities

780-427-7674

This department provides driver assessments to determine driving competence .

DriveAble Testing Locations

780-433-1494 (Edmonton) or 403-252-2243 (Calgary)
Driver assessment program for persons with possible cognitive impairment. Fee for service.

SPECIAL NEEDS

The Support Network-Distress Line

A 24-hour confidential, non-judgmental, supportive, listening service, providing support and referrals for people experiencing difficulty in their lives. Help is also provided in suicide and violent situations.
Edmonton and area, call 780-482-4357 (HELP)
Drayton Valley, High Prairie, and Westview and Aspen Health Authorities regions: 1-800-232-7288

CARING FOR YOURSELF

Calgary Family Resource Centre

403-303-6027
The centre provides caregivers with referral to information and support services. Also offers seminar series called "Taking Care of You."

The Family Centre

780-423-2831
A non-profit centre offering homemaking services for in-home care and appointments. Family counselling and development workshops/seminars and interpreting services offered. Charges a sliding scale fee for services.

Saskatchewan

GOVERNMENT

In Saskatchewan, 32 District Health Boards and one Health Authority in the north are responsible for all health care within the province. They are your first step to finding the services you need in your area. The Health Boards and Health Authority hire their own staff and do not contract work out to independent companies. Phone the Saskatchewan Health and Social Services Department of Community Care at 306-787-1501 for the District Health Board nearest you. Long-term care facilities are also referred through this system.

Information is also available through the Saskatchewan Association of Health Organizations: SAHO Regina: 306-347-5500 SAHO Saskatoon: 306-374-3480 Web: www.saho.org

Saskatchewan has a number of housing programs to assist seniors including:Affordable Housing Rentals (seniors rentals), Home Adaptations for Seniors Independence (HASI), Saskatchewan Assisted Living Services (SALS), and Social Housing Rental Program - Seniors Rentals

For information, call toll-free, 1-800-814-8688 to speak to someone at the nearest Housing Territory Operations office, or go to the web site at www.municipal.gov.sk.ca/housing/programs/shtml.

Aids to Independent Living
306-787-6970
Equipment is available on a loan basis if requisitioned by a designated health professional.

Program Support Unit Community Care Branch — Saskatchewan Health
306-787-1509
www.health.gov.sk.ca

Human Resources Development Canada
For service in English: 1-800-277-9914 in French: 1-800-277-9915
www.sk.hrdc-drhc.gc.ca
HRDC administers two income assistance programs for seniors through its Income Security Programs (CPP & OAS).

Veterans Affairs
306-780-5240, or 1-800-665-3420
For information on Veteran Affairs programs contact the Manitoba district office of Veterans Affairs Canada. Refer to GENERAL RESOURCES in the Canada-wide listings for a description of services offered.

The Canadian Seniors Policies and Programs Database
www.sppd.gc.ca
The SPPD is an Internet based database of government policies and programs for which seniors are the primary beneficiaries. It was developed and is maintained by federal, provincial and territorial governments.

LONG-TERM CARE FACILITIES

There are a number of facilities throughout the province which provide varying levels of care. Your local District Health Board has a complete list. Your care co-ordinator will be able to direct you to the proper facility based on the level of care that your loved one requires.

GENERAL RESOURCES/SPECIAL NEEDS

Alzheimer Society of Saskatchewan

1-800-263-3367

www.alzheimer.sk.ca

Provides educational and support programs to improve awareness and to assist families and individuals coping with the disease; also offers support groups, education sessions, a care-at-home service department that trains nurses, health care aids, etc., for at-home work. All at-home services are fee based and are reviewed on a case-by-case basis to determine eligibility for financial aid.

The Arthritis Society

306-352-3312 or 1-800-321-1433

www.arthritis.ca

A non-profit organization devoted solely to funding and promoting arthritis research, patient care and public education.

Canadian Cancer Society Saskatchewan Division

306-522-7347 or 1-877-977-HOPE

Cancer information services: 1-888-939-3333

www.sk.cancer.ca

Each divisional office provides various kinds of services; call to find out what is available.

The Canadian Deafblind & Rubella Association

306-374-0022

www.cdbra.ca

Provides intervention services to deaf-blind and rubella handicapped people throughout Saskatchewan.

The Canadian Diabetes Association

204-925-3800 or 1-800-BANTING

www.diabetes.ca

A national, independent, self-financing organization, works to improve the quality of life of Canadians affected by diabetes by being the leading force in research, service, advocacy and education.

Canadian National Institute for the Blind — Saskatchewan

306-525-2571

The CNIB offers numerous resources including counselling and referral, orientation and mobility training, sight enhancement, and technical aids.

The Canadian Mental Health Association

306-525-5601

www.cmhask.com

Promotes mental health in Saskatchewan and advocates ensuring the best care, treatment, and rehabilitation for persons with emotional and mental problems.

The Canadian Red Cross Society.

306-721-1600

Emergency 24 hour service 1-888-800-6493

Website: www.redcross.ca

Offers a variety of services to seniors throughout the province.

Heart and Stroke Foundation of Saskatchewan.

306-244-2124

www.heartandstroke.ca

Provides free literature on a wide range of topics such as controlling stress, cholesterol, managing high blood pressure and smoking cessation.

The Multiple Sclerosis Society of Canada.

1-800-268-7582 or 306-522-5600

www.mssociety.ca

Undertakes research into the cause and cure of multiple sclerosis and works to educate the public about the condition.

Saskatchewan Association for Community Living (SACL)

1-800-667-8450

Helps individuals with a developmental disability who are aging. Support services and counselling are based on need.

Saskatchewan Deaf and Hard of Hearing Services Inc.

1-800-565-3323

This non-profit organization serves deaf, hard of hearing, and late-deafened persons with a variety of support services. These include communication services, social work, and hearing aid battery sales.

Saskatchewan Self-Help Network

306-373-8908

SeniorsCan

The SeniorsCan Internet Program is a highly acclaimed guide for retirees and older adults to Canadian and global information and services. www.crm.mb.ca/sk/index.html

NURSING AND HOMEMAKING AGENCIES

For nursing and homemaking agencies in your area, please refer to NURSING AND HOMEMAKING AGENCIES in the Canada-wide listings.

HOME HEALTH CARE RETAILERS, HOME SAFETY, AND ENVIRONMENT

There are a number of home health care retailers located throughout the province that can help you find the right products for your specific needs. To find a store near you, please refer HOME HEALTH CARE RETAILERS, HOME SAFETY, AND ENVIRONMENT in the Canada-wide listings.

FINANCIAL PLANNING/LEGAL

Office of the Public Guardian and Trustee

306-787-5427

This office is responsible for protecting the financial rights of cognitively challenged people. They help individuals make decisions on personal care and medical treatment. The office also advises family members on guardianship and on how to obtain the legal authority to make decisions on behalf of loved ones.

Saskatchewan Legal Aid Commission
306-933-5300
This group provides legal services to people who can't afford a lawyer. Offices are located throughout the province.

VOLUNTEER AGENCIES

TRANSPORTATION

In each province, the Ministry of Transportation makes the official decision on when a person must stop driving.

The family physician is *legally* required to report any case in which someone's driving ability may be impaired due to the progression of age or any resulting condition. The physician must then file his or her report with a Medical Review Board, which may, based on research and interviews with key health care professionals, request a driving assessment to determine driving skills. Based on test results, a decision on whether the individual will be allowed to continue to drive.

If you are concerned about your parents' ability to drive, you can request an independent assessment for one or both of them. Such assessments, which are provided by private companies for a fee, will help you determine your parents' safety while on the road. Contact the Department of Highways and Transportation for more information.

Saskatchewan Department of Highways and Transportation
306-787-4800
This department provides driver assessments to determine driving competence.

Manitoba

GOVERNMENT

The local home care office should be your first point of access in Manitoba. There are a number of home care offices throughout the province. They are all are operated by one of the 12 Regional Health Authorities.

When you contact the local home care office, a health care professional will visit your parents and prepare a report, which will be forwarded to a panel of professionals who will review the application and determine the services and level of care required.

To locate your local home care office, check your local phone directory or call the Winnipeg Regional Health Authority at 204-926-7000.

The Home Care Hotline provides information on a variety of home support services offered through the Manitoba and can be reached at 204-926-8055

The Citizens' Inquiry Service provides direct communication between Manitobans and the provincial government. If you have a question, but are not sure of the appropriate government department or agency to approach, this service will refer you to the correct office; call 1-800-282-8060 or 204-945-3744, or email cis@gov.mb.ca

The Manitoba Seniors Directorate acts as a central point of contact for information and as a liaison with seniors, seniors' organizations and government departments to ensure that government programs, policies and legislation enhance the status of seniors. For more information, call 1-800-665-6565 or 204-945-2127, or go to the web site at www.gov.mb.ca/sd. "Eldercare and You — A Guide for The Eldercaring Employee" is an online publication from the Manitoba Government available at www.gov.mb.ca/sd/eldercare.

The Seniors Abuse Help Line
204-945-1884 or 1-888-896-7183
A confidential information service aimed at providing seniors, caregivers, and others with a one-stop information resource on elder abuse.

Manitoba Health
204-786-7111 or 1-800-378-6699
This provincial office provides information on Regional Health Authorities and can direct you to local services.

Manitoba Health —Continuing Care Department
204-788-6648
This division is responsible for long-term care centres that provide regular treatment services and continuing nursing care.

Pharmacare
204-786-7141 or 1-800-297-8099
www.gov.mb.ca/health/pharmacare
Pharmacare is a drug benefit program for any Manitoban, regardless of age, whose income is seriously affected by high prescription drug costs. Provincial Drug Programs.

Human Resources Development Canada
For service in English: 1-800-277-9914; in French: 1-800-277-9915
www.mb.hrdc-drhc.gc.ca
HRDC administers two income assistance programs for seniors through its Income Security Programs (CPP & OAS).

Veterans Affairs

1-800-665-8717 or 204-983-7040

For information on Veteran Affairs programs contact the Manitoba district office of Veterans Affairs Canada. Refer to GENERAL RESOURCES in the Canada-wide listings for a description of services offered.

The Canadian Seniors Policies and Programs Database

www.sppd.gc.ca

The SPPD is an Internet based database of government policies and programs for which seniors are the primary beneficiaries. It was developed and is maintained by federal, provincial and territorial governments.

LONG-TERM CARE FACILITIES

In Manitoba, there are two types of facilities that provide long-term care: supportive housing and personal care homes. Supportive housing provides light care; personal care homes provide a higher level of care.

An assessment is first conducted by a nurse to determine the person's needs. This assessment is then passed on to a central panel which decides what level of care is required. Based on this decision, a person may be referred to home support, to respite care in the community, or to a long-term care facility.

For more information on assessments, contact your Regional Health Authority or continuing care department at 204-788-6648.

GENERAL RESOURCES/SPECIAL NEEDS

Age and Opportunity

204-956-6440

www.ageopportunity.mb.ca

A community service agency that offers a broad range of services to promote the health and wellness of older adults throughout Winnipeg. In addition, it operates a number of senior centres.

The Alzheimer Society of Manitoba
1-800-378-6699 or 204-943-6622
www.alzheimer.mb.ca
The central part of a volunteer driven, three-tiered structure that links Alzheimer Canada with local Alzheimer groups in various Manitoba communities.

The Arthritis Society
1-800-321-1433 or 204-942-4892
www.arthritis.ca
A non-profit organization devoted solely to funding and promoting arthritis research, patient care and public education.

The Association for Community Living – Manitoba
204-786-1607
Email: aclmb@mb.sympatico.ca
Advocates on behalf of people with mental disabilities to assist them in living a quality lifestyle through the development of community living programs.

Canadian Cancer Society Manitoba Division
1-888-532-6982 or 204-774-7483
www.mb.cancer.ca
Each divisional office provides various kinds of services; call to find out what is available.

Canadian Council of the Blind, Manitoba Division
204-942-8722

The Canadian Deafblind & Rubella Association
Phone 204-949-3730
www.cdbra.ca
Provides intervention services to deaf-blind and rubella handicapped people throughout Manitoba.

The Canadian Diabetes Association,

Phone: 204-925-3800 or 1-800-BANTING

www.diabetes.ca

A national, independent, self-financing organization, works to improve the quality of life of Canadians affected by diabetes by being the leading force in research, service, advocacy and education.

Canadian Hard of Hearing Association — Manitoba branch

204-772-6979

The association provides information and brochures on improving communication skills and helping people deal with hearing loss.

Canadian Mental Health Association

204-775-8888

www.cmhamanitoba.mb.ca

Promotes mental health in Manitoba and advocates ensuring the best care, treatment, and rehabilitation for persons with emotional and mental problems.

Canadian National Institute for the Blind

204-774-5421 or 1-800-552-4893

www.cnib.ca

A charitable, non-profit, voluntary agency that provides rehabilitation and support services to persons who are blind and visually impaired.

The Canadian Red Cross Society

204-982-7330

www.redcross.ca

Offers a variety of services to seniors throughout the province.

Contact Community Information

204-287-8827 or 1-866-266-4636

www.contactmb.org

Email: projectvcw@ mb.sympatico.ca

A community information referral service, which refers Manitobans to social services and programs available through health, educational, cultural and recreational resources in the province.

Heart and Stroke Foundation of Manitoba.

204-949-2000 or 1-888-473-4636

www.heartandstroke.ca

Provides free literature on a wide range of topics such as controlling stress, cholesterol, managing high blood pressure and smoking cessation.

Meals on Wheels

204-956-7711

www3.mb.sympatico.ca/~meals

Provides nutritious meals delivered by volunteers to those in the community unable to prepare or otherwise obtain them.

Multiple Sclerosis Society of Canada

204-943-9595 or 1-800-268-7582

www.mssociety.ca

Undertakes research into the cause and cure of multiple sclerosis and works to educate the public about the condition.

SeniorsCan

www.crm.mb.ca/mb/index.html

The SeniorsCan internet program is a highly acclaimed guide for retirees and older adults to Manitoban, Canadian and global information and services

NURSING AND HOMEMAKING AGENCIES

For nursing and homemaking agencies in your area, please refer to NURSING AND HOMEMAKING AGENCIES in the Canada-wide listings.

HOME HEALTH CARE RETAILERS, HOME SAFETY, AND ENVIRONMENT

There are a number of home health care retailers located throughout the province that can help you find the right products for your specific needs. To find a store near you, please refer HOME HEALTH CARE RETAILERS, HOME SAFETY, AND ENVIRONMENT in the Canada-wide listings.

FINANCIAL PLANNING/LEGAL

ABC's of Fraud Program
204-956-6440
This program gives group presentations to educate seniors about fraud. They distribute complimentary support materials and provide referrals to additional resources.

Legal Aid Manitoba
204-985-8500
Legal Aid Manitoba can fully or partially fund a lawyer to represent a person or group in a lawsuit. Individuals must complete an application and be found eligible. Legal Aid also offers informal drop-in services for simpler questions.

Office of the Public Guardian and Trustee
204-945-2703
This office is responsible for protecting the financial rights of cognitively challenged people. They help individuals make decisions on personal care and medical treatment. The office also advises family members on guardianship and on how to obtain the legal authority to make decisions on behalf of loved ones.

TRANSPORTATION

In each province, the Department of Highways and Transportation makes the official decision on when a person must stop driving. The family physician is *legally* required to report any case in which someone's driving ability may be impaired due to the progression of age or any resulting condition. The physician must file his or her report with a Medical Review Board, which may, based on research and interviews with key health care professionals, request a driving assessment to determine driving skills. Based on test results, a decision will be made on whether the individual will be allowed to continue to drive.

If you are concerned about your parents' ability to drive, you can request an independent assessment for one or both of them. Such assessments, which are provided by private companies for a fee, will help you determine your parents' safety while on the road. Contact the department listed below for more information.

Manitoba Highways and Government Resources Services —
Medical Review Section
204-945-7386
This department provides driver assessments to determine driving competence.

Creative Retirement Manitoba
204-949-2565
www.crm.mb.ca/crm
Email: denesiuk@crm.mb.ca
Offers a number of programs and services for seniors including Fully Alive and the 55 Alive/Mature Driving course.

Ontario

GOVERNMENT

Forty-three Community Care Access Centres (CCAC) located throughout the province serve as the entry point to the Ontario community health care system. The local CCAC will conduct an assessment, and then based on the results, will direct you and your parents to the resources and services that are required.

In addition, you may be able to access private services (such as a nursing or a homemaking agency) from independent associations and organizations through the local CCAC. The centre also will provide you with information on other important caregiving resources such as support groups, crisis lines, related health care associations, and long-term care facilities.

To locate the Community Care Access Centre in your area, call 1-800-268-1154 or visit the web site at www.oaccac.on.ca

Assistive Devices and Home Oxygen Programs
1-800-268-6021 (voice) or
These programs offer financial assistance for those who have a prescribed need for home care products such as wheelchairs, scooters, walkers, etc. They also provide home oxygen services.

Information and Referral Service for Vulnerable Adults and Seniors
416-482-4359, 1-800-665-9092, or 1-800-387-5559

Free telephone referral service that provides information to persons with disabilities including Alzheimer's or dementia.

Ministry of Health and Long Term Care: Health Information Centre
1-800-268-1154

www.gov.on.ca/health

This provincial office is responsible for health care delivery within Ontario. The ministry provides referrals to provincial services (including Community Care Access Centres) that offer specific assistance for different kinds of needs.

Ontario Seniors' Secretariat
1-888-910-1999

www.gov.on.ca/mczcr/seniors

Provides access a variety of information of interest to seniors, their families and those who work with seniors.

Human Resources Development Canada
For service in English: 1-800-277-9914; in French: 1-800-277-9915

www.on.hrdc-drhc.gc.ca

HRDC administers two income assistance programs for seniors through its Income Security Programs (CPP & OAS).

Veterans Affairs
1-800-387-0930

www.vac-acc.gc.ca

For information on Veteran Affairs programs contact the Manitoba district office of Veterans Affairs Canada. Refer to GENERAL RESOURCES in the Canada-wide listings for a description of services offered.

The Canadian Seniors Policies and Programs Database
www.sppd.gc.ca

The SPPD is an Internet based database of government policies and programs for which seniors are the primary beneficiaries. It was developed and is maintained by federal, provincial and territorial governments.

LONG-TERM CARE FACILITIES

There are a number of long-term care facilities throughout the province which provide varying levels of care. Your local Community Care Access Centre has a complete list of local facilities. Your care co-ordinator will be able to direct you to the proper facility based on the level of care that your loved one requires.

In addition, there are numerous retirement homes that provide light, supportive care. The association listed below will help you find the proper facility.

Ontario Residential Care Association (ORCA)

1-800-361-7254 or 905-403-0500

A voluntary, self-regulating organization representing over 250 retirement homes caring for more than 17,000 residents. ORCA operates a consumer information service and publishes a free consumer directory of member facilities.

The Care Guide

www.thecareguide.com

Operated by CARE Planning Partners Inc. of Toronto, this site provides information on seniors' housing and care services. The site features provider search tools, community bulletin boards and an online assessment tool.

GENERAL RESOURCES/SPECIAL NEEDS

Alzheimer Society of Ontario

416-967-5900

www.alzheimer.on.ca

The Alzheimer Society provides educational and support programs to improve awareness and to assist families and individuals coping with the disease; also provides support groups, education sessions, and guest speakers.

The Arthritis Society
416-979-7228 or 1-800-321-1433
www.arthritis.ca
A non-profit organization devoted solely to funding and promoting arthritis research, patient care and public education.

Canadian Cancer Society Ontario Division
Telephone 416-488-5400 or 1-800-268-8874
www.ontario.cancer.ca
Each divisional office provides various kinds of services; call to find out what is available.

The Canadian Deafblind & Rubella Association
519-759-0520 or 1-877-760-7439
www.cdbra.ca
Provides intervention services to deaf-blind and rubella handicapped people throughout Ontario.

The Canadian Diabetes Association
416-363-3373 or 1-800-BANTING
www.diabetes.ca
A national, independent, self-financing organization, works to improve the quality of life of Canadians affected by diabetes by being the leading force in research, service, advocacy and education.

Canadian Hard of Hearing Association — Ontario branch
416-237-1274
The association provides information and brochures on improving communication skills and helping people deal with hearing loss.

Canadian National Institute for the Blind (CNIB)– Ontario
416-413-9480
The CNIB offers numerous resources including counselling and referral, orientation and mobility training, sight enhancement, and technical aids.

The Canadian Mental Health Association
416-977-5580: www.ontario.cmha.ca
Email: division@ontario.cmha.ca
Promotes mental health in Ontario and advocates ensuring the best care, treatment, and rehabilitation for persons with emotional and mental problems.

The Canadian Red Cross Society
905-890-1000
Website: www.redcross.ca
Offers a variety of services to seniors throughout the province.

Consumer Health Information Service (CHIS)
1-800-667-1999 (outside Toronto) or 416-393-7056 (in Toronto)
CHIS provides names of relevant associations and resources as a starting point and mails out custom packages of helpful information for consumers to make more informed decisions about their own health care.

Heart and Stroke Foundation of Ontario
416-489-7100
www.heartandstroke.ca
Provides free literature on a wide range of topics such as controlling stress, cholesterol, managing high blood pressure and smoking cessation.

Seniors for Seniors
416-481-2733
Provides drop-in senior companions for various services, including overnight and 24-hour live-in support in the Golden Horseshoe area. Fee for service.

SeniorsCan
www.crm.on.ca/index.html
The SeniorsCan Internet Program is a highly acclaimed guide for retirees and older adults to Canadian and global information and services.

NURSING AND HOMEMAKING AGENCIES

Ontario Home Health Care Providers Association
Web: www.ohhcpa.on.ca
Representing a number of organizations.

St. Elizabeth Health Care
905-940-9655
www.saintelizabeth.com
A non-profit nursing agency with a full range of nursing and home-making services.

For other nursing and homemaking agencies in your area, please refer to NURSING AND HOMEMAKING AGENCIES in the Canada-wide listings.

HOME HEALTH CARE RETAILERS, HOME SAFETY, AND ENVIRONMENT

There are a number of home health care stores located throughout the province that can help you find the right products for your specific needs. To find a store near you, please refer to HOME HEALTH CARE RETAILERS, HOME SAFETY, AND ENVIRONMENT in the Canada-wide listings.

FINANCIAL PLANNING/LEGAL

ABC's of Fraud Program
416-961-6888
This program uses group presentations to educate seniors about fraud. They distribute complimentary support materials and referrals to additional resources.

Advocacy Centre for the Elderly (ACE)

416-598-2656

A legal clinic for low-income, 60+ seniors in the Greater Toronto area. ACE offers one-on-one legal advice and provides updates on new legislation relevant to the rights of seniors. Most of the ACE services are provided free of charge.

Dial-A-Law: The Law Society of Upper Canada

416-947-3330, or 1-800-268-8326

Lawyer referral service that provides a complimentary half-hour of initial legal counselling. However, callers must dial 1-900-565-4577 and pay $6 per call.

Legal Aid Ontario

416-979-1446

Legal Aid is available to lower-income people for a variety of legal issues. Eligibility is based on financial need and the type of case. The applicant may pay nothing or a portion of the costs of the legal aid, depending on his or her financial situation. Once approved, a legal aid certificate entitles a person to retain the lawyer of his or her choice. The lawyer is then reimbursed by Legal Aid Ontario.

Office of the Public Guardian and Trustee

416-314-2800

This office is responsible for protecting the financial rights of cognitively challenged people. They help individuals make decisions on personal care and medical treatment. The office also advises family members on guardianship and on how to obtain the legal authority to make decisions on behalf of loved ones.

TRANSPORTATION

In each province, the Ministry of Transportation makes the official decision on when a person with dementia must stop driving. The family physician is *legally* required to report any case in which someone's driving ability may be impaired due to age or any resulting condition. The physician must file his or her report with a Medical Review Board, which may, based on research and interviews with key health care professionals, request a driving assessment to determine driving skills. Based on test results, a decision will be made on whether the individual will be allowed to continue to drive.

If you are concerned about your parents' ability to drive, you can request an independent assessment for one or both of them Such assessments, which are provided by private companies for a fee, will help you determine your parents' safety while on the road.

Ontario Ministry of Transportation
416-235-4686
This department provides driver assessments to determine driving competency.

DriveAble Testing Locations
416-498-6429
Driver assessment program. Fee for service.

CARING FOR YOURSELF

Self Help Resource Centre
1-888-283-8806
www.selfhelp.on.ca
This centre provides listings of self-help groups across Ontario for family, friends, and caregivers looking after ageing parents, and many other self-help categories.

Ontario Community Support Association
1-800-267-6272
www.ocsa.on.ca
A good resource to connect to some 360 agencies across Ontario providing a host of services including Meals on Wheels, many of which will be relevant to caregivers, including referrals to organizations that offer therapeutic counselling and relief from caregiving duties.

Quebec

PROVINCIAL GOVERNMENT

The Quebec government has a very centralized approach to providing information about its services. Communication-Québec is its principal information arm, providing comprehensive lists and descriptions of services available. Call 1-800-363-1363, or visit the website at www.comm-gc.gouv.qc.ca/en/guides_55over.html and download the English pdf file with extensive listings.

Centres Locaux de Service Communitaires (CLSCs) are located throughout the province and are your first contact for finding the health care services you need. Each CLSC provides a number of services, including nursing care, home care and domestic help, and referrals to outside agencies, associations, and volunteer groups.

You can find the closest CLSC by calling the Association des CLSC at 514-931-1448, or by visiting the Ministère de la Santé et des Services Sociaux website at www.msss.gouv.qc.ca and entering your postal code.

LONG-TERM CARE FACILITIES

There are a number of facilities throughout the province which provide varying levels of care. Your local CLSC has a complete list. Your care co-ordinator will be able to direct you to the proper facility based on the level of care that your parent requires.

GENERAL RESOURCES

Fédération Québécoise Sociétés Alzheimers
(Federation of Quebec Alzheimers Societies)
1-888-636-6437

The Alzheimer's Society provides educational and support programs to improve awareness and to assist families and individuals coping with the disease and will refer callers to regional offices of the Alzheimer's Society that, in turn, will provide a variety of services for caregivers of persons with dementia or Alzheimer's.

Canadian Cancer Society — Quebec Division
514-255-5151

www.quebec.cancer.ca/eng

Each divisional office provides various kinds of support and services; call to find out what is available.

Canadian Arthritis Society
1-800-321-1433

www.arthritis.ca

A non-profit organization devoted solely to funding and promoting arthritis research, patient care, and public education.

Canadian Liver Foundation
514-876-4171 or 1-800-563-5483

www.liver.ca

Non-profit organization devoted to liver illnesses.

Héma Québec

1-888-646-2237

www.hema-quebec.ca

The Quebec equivalent of the Red Cross Blood Services.

FINANCIAL PLANNING/LEGAL

Curateur public du Quebec (Public Trustee)

514-873-4074

This office is responsible for protecting the financial rights of cognitively challenged people. They help individuals make decisions on personal care and medical treatment, offers power of attorney kits and wills, and help search for heirs and next-of-kin. The office also advises family members on guardianship and how to obtain the legal authority to make decisions on behalf of loved ones.

Commission des services juridiques (Legal Aid)

514-873-3562

Legal Aid offers economically disadvantaged people access to the courts, the professional services of an attorney or a notary, and the information they need regarding their rights and obligations. Eligibility for legal aid is based on several factors including the applicant's family obligations, income, property, and liquid assets.

Persons eligible are entitled to the services of a legal aid lawyer. They are also entitled to a lawyer in private practice if he or she accepts; however, not all services are covered.

TRANSPORTATION

In each province, the Ministry of Transportation makes the official decision on when a person must stop driving. The family physician is *legally* required to report any case in which driving ability may be impaired due to the progression of age or any resulting condition. The physician must then file his or her report with a Medical Review Board, which may, based on research and interviews with key health care professionals, request a driving assessment to determine driving skills. Based on test results, a decision will be made on whether the individual is allowed to continue to drive.

If you are concerned about your parents' ability to drive, you can request an independent assessment for one or both of them. Such assessments, which are provided by private companies for a fee, will help you determine your parents' safety while on the road.

Ministère des Transports du Québec
418-643-6864
This department provides driver assessments to determine driving competence.

DriveAble Testing
514-733-1414
Driver assessment program. Fee for service.

SPECIAL NEEDS

Canadian Hard of Hearing Association — Quebec branch
613-526-1584
This association provides information and brochures on improving communication skills and helping people deal with hearing loss.

New Brunswick

GOVERNMENT

In New Brunswick, the home and community health care services are offered through the <u>Department of Family and Community Service</u> regional offices. Each office will conduct an assessment and financial evaluation to determine the level of care required. Based upon this evaluation, you will then be referred to the correct services your parents require. Whenever possible, individuals are expected to contribute financially to their care. To locate a Family and Community Service office near you, call 1-888-762-8600.

Within government, the Office for Family and Prevention Services provides a focus for seniors' issues. The Office also works in partnership with community groups in program development; for more information, call 506-453-2950.

The third edition of the <u>Seniors' Guide to Services and Programs</u> is available on the Internet at www. gnb.ca/Fcs-sfc/Seniors/introe.html

<u>Providing Care and Assistance to Older Family Members</u> is another helpful publication available at www.gnb.ca/Fcs-sfc/Senior/hints.html

Family and Community Social Services

506-453-2001

www.gnb.ca/0017/index-e.asp

This department offers long-term and in-home support services based on assessments and eligibility (depends on the level of needs of the individual). Also provides case management and referrals to various service providers. The web site also has a very practical section on hints for caregivers.

Prescription Drug Program

506-867-4515 or 1-800-332-3692

Provides prescription drug benefits to eligible residents of New Brunswick. The program is targeted to those with a demonstrated medical and financial need.

Veterans Affairs

Campbellton District Office

Telephone: (506) 789-4700 or1-800-350-7955

Saint John District Office

Telephone: (506) 636-4815 or1-800-349-9788

For information on Veteran Affairs programs, contact one of the New Brunswick district offices of Veterans Affairs Canada.

Human Resources Development Canada

For service in English: 1-800-277-9914;

in French: 1-800-277-9915

www.nb.hrdc-drhc.gc.ca

Email: isp-psr.mail-poste@hrdc-drhc.gc.ca

HRDC administers two income assistance programs for seniors through its Income Security Programs (CPP & OAS).

The Canadian Seniors Policies and Programs Database

http://www.sppd.gc.ca

The SPPD is an Internet based database of government policies and programs for which seniors are the primary beneficiaries. It was developed and is maintained by federal, provincial and territorial governments.

LONG-TERM CARE FACILITIES

In New Brunswick, there are two types of long-term care facilities: special care homes and nursing homes. Special care homes are for people who can care for themselves; nursing homes provide a higher level of support and are for people who require 24-hour care.

Admission to both is based on a referral from a family physician or by contacting the Department of Family and Community Services (see PROVINCIAL GOVERNMENT above) to obtain information and start the process. Either requires an assessment conducted by a public health nurse or social worker to determine the level of care required, funding required, and any other needs. Admission is based on the assessment.

GENERAL RESOURCES/ SPECIAL NEEDS

Alzheimer Society of New Brunswick
506-459-4280
www.alzheimer.nb.ca
Family Information and Referral Line 1-800-664-8411
This organization is the central part of a volunteer driven, three-tiered structure that links Alzheimer Canada with local Alzheimer groups in various New Brunswick communities

Arthritis Society New Brunswick Division
506-4527191 or 1-800-321-1433
www.arthritis.ca
A non-profit organization devoted solely to funding and promoting arthritis research, patient care and public education.

The Blue Cross Seniors' Health Program
1-800-565-0065
Provides access to the New Brunswick Drug Program for those residents of the province who are not otherwise eligible.

Canadian Cancer Society New Brunswick Division

506-634-6272

www.nb. cancer.ca

E-mail: ccsnb@nbnet.nb.ca

Each divisional office provides various services; call to find out what is available.

Canadian Deafblind & Rubella Association.

506-452-1544

Provides intervention services to deaf-blind and rubella handicapped people throughout New Brunswick and Prince Edward Island.

Canadian Diabetes Association,

506-452-9009 or 1-800-884-4232

A national, independent, self-financing organization, works to improve the quality of life of Canadians affected by diabetes by being the leading force in research, service, advocacy and education.

Canadian Council of the Blind

506-789-1710

Canadian Hard of Hearing Association — New Brunswick branch

506-859-6930

Provides information and brochures on improving communication skills and helping people deal with hearing loss.

Canadian Mental Health Association

506-455-5231

Promotes mental health in New Brunswick and advocates ensuring the best care, treatment, and rehabilitation for persons with emotional and mental problems.

Canadian National Institute for the Blind

506-458-0060

A charitable, non-profit, voluntary agency that provides rehabilitation and support services to persons who are blind and visually impaired.

Canadian Red Cross Society
506-648-5000
Offers a variety of services to seniors throughout the province including homecare, meals-on-wheels, equipment loan programs and a unique home partner program.

Canadian Rehabilitation Council for the Disabled— New Brunswick Branch
506-458-8739
Helps people of all ages who may have physical disabilities achieve maximum rehabilitation.

Heart and Stroke Foundation of New Brunswick
(506) 634-1620 or 1-800-663-3600
Provides free literature on a wide range of topics such as controlling stress, cholesterol, managing high blood pressure and smoking cessation.

New Brunswick Senior Citizen's Federation
506-857-8242 or 1-800-453-4333 or
Strives for awareness of the human community and its environment by exploring issues relevant to seniors.

The Multiple Sclerosis Society of Canada
902-468-8230
Undertakes research into the cause and cure of multiple sclerosis and works to educate the public about the condition.

New Brunswick Association for Community Living
505-458-8866
Non-profit provincial federation of 26 local associations located through-out the province.

Chimo Crisis Line
1-800-667-5005
A toll-free, 24 hours a day, province-wide telephone helpline for people who are experiencing a crisis.

Tele-Care

1-800-244-8353

A bilingual, province-wide 24-hour service, for help with non-emergency medical problems

NURSING AND HOMEMAKING AGENCIES

For nursing and homemaking agencies in your area, please refer to NURSING AND HOMEMAKING AGENCIES in the Canada-wide listings.

HOME HEALTH CARE RETAILERS, HOME SAFETY, AND ENVIRONMENT

There are a number of home health care retailers located throughout the province that can help you find the right products for your specific needs. To find a store near you, please refer to HOME HEALTH CARE RETAILERS, HOME SAFETY, AND ENVIRONMENT in the Canada-wide listings.

VOLUNTEER AGENCIES

TRANSPORTATION

In each province, the Ministry of Transportation makes the official decision on when a person with dementia must stop driving.

The family physician is legally required to report any case in which driving ability may be impaired due to the progression of age or any resulting condition. The physician must file his or her report with a Medical Review Board, which may, based on research and interviews with key health care professionals, request a driving assessment to determine driving skills. Based on test results, a decision will be made on whether the individual will be allowed to continue to drive.

If you are concerned about your parents' ability to drive, you can request an independent assessment for one or both of them. Such assessments, which are provided by private companies for a fee, will help you determine your parents' safety while on the road. Contact the department below for more information.

New Brunswick Department of Transportation
506-453-3939

This department provides driver assessments to determine driving competence.

Vehicle Retrofitting and Accessible Vehicle Program
506-453-2802

This program is designed to provide assistance for retrofitting vehicles with eligible accessibility feature

Nova Scotia

GOVERNMENT

Public Enquiries Officers respond to telephone enquiries about all provincial government services, programs and initiatives. The service offers a province-wide toll-free telephone line at 1-800-670-4357; the local number is 902-424-5200.

Health care service delivery is provided through one of nine District Health Authorities. Each is responsible for delivering all care services to people in its particular region. In addition, the Nova Scotia Department of Health will be establishing a toll-free number that will direct you to the closest facility.

Call the Nova Scotia Department of Health at 1-800-565-3611 and leave a message - a government representative will respond to your message and help direct you to the proper services.

The province is in the pilot stage of a single entry access program on the Internet. For the most current information go to www.gov.ns.ca/health/sea

Nova Scotia Department of Health: Home Care Department

1-800-225-7225 or 902-424-4653 (toll free within the province that will direct the caller to the nearest Home Care branch).

This office provides home care services based on the individual's needs, including home oxygen service, family relief, nursing services, case management, and more. Nursing services are free. There may be a fee, based on the individual's income, for other services (e.g., oxygen and home support).

Nova Scotia Department of Health: Long-Term Care Program

902-424-4476

This department provides information and referrals to long -term care facilities, such as a nursing or retirement home. An assessment is first conducted to determine the individual's level of care.

Senior Citizens' Secretariat and Seniors Information Line

1-800-670-0065 (424-0065 for Halifax/Dartmouth)

www.gov.ns.ca/health/seniors/senior1.htm

A comprehensive listing of provincial government services for seniors. The publication Programs For Seniors is updated annually and is available online or as a booklet.

Human Resources Development Canada

For service in English: 1-800-277-9914;

in French: 1-800-277-9915www.ns.hrdc-drhc.gc.ca

Email: isp-psr.mail-poste@hrdc-drhc.gc.ca

HRDC administers two income assistance programs for seniors through its Income Security Programs (CPP & OAS).

Veterans Affairs

For information on Veteran Affairs programs contact the Manitoba district office of Veterans Affairs Canada. Refer to GENERAL RESOURCES in the Canada-wide listings for a description of services offered.

902-426-6448 or 1-800-565-1528

The Canadian Seniors Policies and Programs Database

www.sppd.gc.ca

The SPPD is an Internet based database of government policies and programs for which seniors are the primary beneficiaries. It was developed and is maintained by federal, provincial and territorial governments.

LONG-TERM CARE FACILITIES

There are a number of facilities throughout the province that provide varying levels of care. Your local District Health Authority has a complete list. Your care co-ordinator will be able to direct you to the proper facility based on the level of care that your parent requires. For more information about home care and lont-term care services, call 1-800-225-7225.

GENERAL RESOURCES/SPECIAL NEEDS

Alzheimer Society of Nova Scotia
902-422-7961
www.alzheimer.ns.ca
The Alzheimer Society provides educational and support programs to improve awareness and to assist families and individuals coping with the disease; information on books and resources, phone support, guest speakers, support groups, community resources, and a number of innovative programs throughout the province. One program is an eight-week course administered through the QE II Hospital which deals with overall caregiving issues for persons in the early stages of dementia.

Arthritis Society
902-429-7025 or 1-800-321-1433
www.arthritis.ca
A non-profit organization devoted solely to funding and promoting arthritis research, patient care and public education.

Canadian Cancer Society Nova Scotia Division
902-423-6183 or 1-800-639-0222
www.cancer.ca

Each divisional office provides various services; call to find out what is available.

Canadian Diabetes Association

902-453-4CDA (4232), or 1-800-326-7712

www.diabetes.ca

A national, independent, self-financing organization, works to improve the quality of life of Canadians affected by diabetes by being the leading force in research, service, advocacy and education.

Canadian Mental Health Association

902-466-6600

www.cmhans.org

Promotes mental health in Nova Scotia and advocates ensuring the best care, treatment, and rehabilitation for persons with emotional and mental problems.

Canadian National Institute for the Blind (CNIB) – Nova Scotia

902-453-1480 or 1-800-565-5147

www.cnib.ca

The CNIB offers numerous resources including counselling and referral, orientation and mobility training, sight enhancement, and technical aids.

Canadian Red Cross Society

902-423-3680

www.redcross.ca

Offers a variety of services to seniors throughout the province

Caregiver Resource Centre Library

902-457-6561

Over 1,000 books, videos, and other resources available to lend free of charge to caregivers for the elderly. Affiliated with the Nova Scotia Centre on Aging.

Continuing Care Association of Nova Scotia (CCANS)

902-453-2977

www.ccans.cjb.net

CCANS is a not-for-profit organization representing some 50 facilities and service providers that offer residential care or various support services for the elderly with special needs.

Heart and Stroke Foundation of Nova Scotia.

902-423-7530

www.heartandstroke.ca

Provides free literature on a wide range of topics such as controlling stress, cholesterol, managing high blood pressure and smoking cessation

Late-Deafened Adult Support Group

902-434-1673

Provides emotional support and resources to residents in the Halifax area.

Society of Deaf and Hard of Hearing Nova Scotians

902-422-7130

Assists adult deaf, deafened, and hard of hearing Nova Scotians to gain access to existing public, private, and community services.

Multiple Sclerosis Society of Canada

1-800-268-7582

www.mssociety.ca

E-mail:info.atlantic@mssociety.ca

Undertakes research into the cause and cure of multiple sclerosis and works to educate the public about the condition.

Nova Scotia Association of Health Organizations (NSAHO)

902-832-8500

www.nsaho.ns.ca

Represents more than 100 organizations, including nine district health authorities, 50 continuing care providers, and home care and home support agencies.

SeniorsCan

www.crm.ns.ca/index/html

The SeniorsCan Internet Program is a highly acclaimed guide for retirees and older adults to Canadian and global information and services.

NURSING AND HOMEMAKING AGENCIES

For nursing and homemaking agencies in your area, please refer to NURSING AND HOMEMAKING AGENCIES in the Canada-wide listings.

HOME HEALTH CARE RETAILERS, HOME SAFETY, AND ENVIRONMENT

There are a number of home health care retailers located throughout the province that can help you find the right products for your specific needs. To find a store near you, please refer HOME HEALTH CARE RETAILERS, HOME SAFETY, AND ENVIRONMENT in the Canada-wide listings.

FINANCIAL PLANNING/LEGAL

Legal Information Society of Nova Scotia

902-454-2198

Provides information and resources about wills, family, power of attorney, and other legal matters.

Nova Scotia Legal Aid

902-420-3471

There are 13 regional offices and three sub-offices in the province. Legal aid may be provided to people on social assistance or in an equivalent financial position in certain areas of family and criminal law.

Public Trustee of Nova Scotia

902-424-7760

This office is responsible for protecting the financial rights of cognitively challenged people. They help individuals make decisions on personal care and medical treatment. The office also advises family members on guardianship and on how to obtain the legal authority to make decisions on behalf of loved ones.

VOLUNTEER AGENCIES

Good Neighbours.
902-424-0065 or 1-800-670-0065
Promotes an attitude to encourage people to reach out and help one another and to create caring, sharing and friendly communities.

Family Caregivers Association of Nova Scotia
902-421-7390 or 1-877-488-7390
Non-profit association that offers services for all caregivers. Provides newsletter and other resources. Has a strong network with other caregiving groups throughout the province.

The Seniors' Goodwill Ambassador Program
902-424-4737 or 1-800-670-0065
Part of a government project initiated in order to promote Nova Scotia at home and abroad by utilizing the skills of volunteers 50 years of age and older.

Volunteer Resource Centre - Sydney
902-562-1245
Coordinates and administers: Meals on Wheels, Each One Teach One, a friendly visiting service, transportation, and snow shovelling. It is a non-profit organization and a member of the United Way of Cape Breton.

TRANSPORTATION

In each province, the Ministry of Transportation makes the official deci-

RESOURCE GUIDE: *Nova Scotia*

sion on when a person must stop driving. The family physician is *legally* required to report any cases in which driving ability may be impaired due to the progression of age or any resulting condition. The physician must then file his or her report with a Medical Review Board, which may, based on research and interviews with key health care professionals, request a driving assessment to determine driving skills. Based on test results, a decision will be made on whether the individual will be allowed to continue to drive.

If you are concerned about your parents' ability to drive, you can request an independent assessment for each or both of them. Such assessments, which are provided by private companies for a fee, will help you determine your parents' safety while on the road. Contact the department below for more information.

Registry of Motor Vehicles: Medical Section
902-424-5732
This department provides driver assessments to determine driving competence.

Nova Scotia Safety Council 55 Alive
902-454-9621
A national mature driver refresher course. The course consists of 6 hours of classroom instruction only, commonly offered over two mornings. There are no tests or any negative effect on the license.

Prince Edward Island

PROVINCIAL GOVERNMENT

In PEI, you will be conected with a health professional who will assist you in exploring options for care. Each region has a Home Care Office that offers a variety of services.

Upon contacting the local office, a health care professional will visit your home and conduct an assessment. This assessment will help the professional to determine your parent's needs and the level of care that he or she requires.

To locate your local Home Care Office, check your local phone directory, or go to the comprehensive provincial website at www.gov.pe.ca/seniors. Another very good resource is the province-wiede Health Information Resource Centre; call 1-800-241-6970, or visit www.hirc.pe.ca. As well, a helpful Directory of Self-Help Groups and Community Resources is available at 1-800-682-1648.

PEI Department of Health and Social Services
902-368-6190
This department provides information on provincial health services and departments related to home care.

Human Resources Development Canada

For service in English: 1-800-277-9914; in French: 1-800-277-9915

www.pe.hrdc-drhc.gc.ca

Email: isp-psr.mail-poste@hrdc-drhc.gc.ca

HRDC administers two income assistance programs for seniors through its Income Security Programs (CPP & OAS).

Veterans Affairs

For information on Veteran Affairs programs contact the PEI district office of Veterans Affairs Canada. Refer to GENERAL RESOURCES in the Canada-wide listings for a description of services offered.

902-566-8677 or 1-800-565-2422

The Canadian Seniors Policies and Programs Database

www.sppd.gc.ca

The SPPD is an Internet based database of government policies and programs for which seniors are the primary beneficiaries. It was developed and is maintained by federal, provincial and territorial governments.

LONG-TERM CARE FACILITIES

Nursing care is accessed by contacting a placement officer in one of the five health regions on PEI. There are a number of facilities throughout the province that provide varying levels of care. Your local Home Care Office has a complete list. Your care co-ordinator will be able to direct you to the proper facility based on the level of care that your loved one requires.

GENERAL RESOURCES/SPECIAL NEEDS

Alzheimer Society of PEI

902-628-2257

The Alzheimer Society provides educational and support programs to improve awareness and to assist families and individuals coping with the disease, as well as information on books, and resources, phone support, guest speakers, support groups, community resources, and a number of innovative programs throughout the province.

Arthritis Society

902-628-2288 or 1-800-321-1433

www.arthritis.ca

A non-profit organization devoted solely to funding and promoting arthritis research, patient care and public education.

Canadian Cancer Society PEI Division

902-566-4007 or 1-866-566-4007

www.pei.cancer.ca

Canadian Diabetes Association

902-894-3005 or 1-800-BANTING (1-800-226-8464)

www.diabetes.ca

A national, independent, self-financing organization, works to improve the quality of life of Canadians affected by diabetes by being the leading force in research, service, advocacy and education.

Canadian Mental Health Association.

902-566-3034

www.cmha.pe.ca

Promotes mental health in PEI and advocates ensuring the best care, treatment, and rehabilitation for persons with emotional and mental problems

Canadian National Institute for the Blind .

902-566-2580

www.cnib.ca

A charitable, non-profit, voluntary agency that provides rehabilitation and support services to persons who are blind and visually impaired.

Canadian Red Cross Society

902-628-6262

www.redcross.ca

Offers a variety of services to seniors throughout the province.

Heart and Stroke Foundation of PEI

902-892-7441

www.heartandstroke.ca

Provides free literature on a wide range of topics such as controlling stress, cholesterol, managing high blood pressure and smoking cessation.

Island Help Line

1-800-218-2885

Multiple Sclerosis Society of Canada

902-468-8230 or 1-800-268-7582

www.mssociety.ca

Undertakes research into the cause and cure of multiple sclerosis and works to educate the public about the condition.

Prince Edward Island Association for the Hearing Impaired

902-892-6585

Provides services and information for the hearing impaired in PEI.

Seniors Info Line.

902-368-7538

Provides access to information about services that support seniors in their wish to remain in their own homes as long as possible

SeniorsCan

www.crm.pei.ca/index.html

The SeniorsCan Internet Program is a highly acclaimed guide for retirees and older adults to Canadian and global information and services.

NURSING AND HOMEMAKING AGENCIES

For nursing and homemaking agencies in your area, please refer to NURSING AND HOMEMAKING AGENCIES in the Canada-wide listings.

HOME HEALTH CARE RETAILERS, HOME SAFETY, AND ENVIRONMENT

There are a number of home health care retailers located throughout the province that can help you find the right products for your specific needs. To find a store near you, please refer to HOME HEALTH CARE RETAILERS, HOME SAFETY, AND ENVIRONMENT in the Canada-wide listings.

FINANCIAL PLANNING/LEGAL

Office of the Public Guardian and Trustee
902-368-4564
This office is responsible for protecting the financial rights of cognitively challenged people. They help individuals make decisions on personal care and medical treatment. The office also advises family members on guardianship and on how to obtain the legal authority to make decisions on behalf of loved ones.

TRANSPORTATION

In each province, the Ministry of Transportation makes the official decision on when a person must stop driving. The family physician is ethically required to report any case in which someone's driving ability may be impaired due to the progression of age or any resulting condition. The physician must file his or her report with a Medical Review Board, which may based on research and interviews with key health care professionals, request a driving assessment to determine driving skills. Based on test results, a decision will be made on whether the individual will be allowed to continue to drive.

If you are concerned about your parents' ability to drive, you can request an independent assessment for one or both of them. Such assessments, which are provided by private companies for a fee, will help you determine your parents' safety while on the road. Contact the department below for more information.

PEI Transportation and Public Works
902-368-5100
This department provides driver assessments to determine driving competence.

PEI Safety Council offers the 55 Alive seniors driving course.
1-800-618-4697

Newfoundland and Labrador

GOVERNMENT

There are six regional Community Health Boards in Newfoundland that look after home care and other related services for aging parents with special needs.

Once you contact the local office, a health care professional will visit your parent and conduct an assessment. This assessment will help determine your parent's needs and the level of care that he or she may require.

Call the Department of Health and Community Services at 709-729-5021 to locate the office nearest to you.

LONG-TERM CARE FACILITIES

There are a number of facilities throughout the province that provide varying levels of care. Your local Community Health Board has a complete list. Your care co-ordinator will be able to direct you to the proper facility based on the level of care that your parent requires.

GENERAL RESOURCES

Alzheimer Society of Newfoundland and Labrador
709-576-0608

The Alzheimer Society provides educational and support programs to improve awareness and to assist families and individuals coping with the diseas,as well as information on books and resources, phone support, guest speakers, support groups, community resources, and a number of innovative programs throughout the province.

Seniors' Resource Centre
709-737-2333 or 1-800-563-5599

The centre offers a number of programs for caregivers including a free newsletter and a Friday friendship club, as well as friendly visiting and other community services. Operates a toll-free line for unpaid caregivers at 1-888-571-2273.

Veterans Affairs District Office
709-772-4716 or 1-800-563-9623

Please refer to GENERAL RESOURCES in the Canada-wide listings for a description of services offered.

NURSING AND HOMEMAKING AGENCIES

For nursing and homemaking agencies in your area, please refer to NURSING AND HOMEMAKING AGENCIES in the Canada-wide listings.

HOME HEALTH CARE RETAILERS, HOME SAFETY, AND ENVIRONMENT

There are a number of home health care retailers located throughout the province that can help you find the right products for your specific needs. To find a store near you, please refer to HOME HEALTH CARE RETAILERS, HOME SAFETY, AND ENVIRONMENT in the

Canada-wide listings.

FINANCIAL PLANNING/LEGAL

ABC's of Fraud Program
709-737-2333
This program uses group presentations to educate seniors about fraud. They distribute complimentary support materials and offer referrals to additional resources.

Office of the Public Guardian and Trustee
709-729-4504
This office is responsible for protecting the financial rights of cognitively challenged people. They help individuals make decisions on personal care and medical treatment. The office also advises family members on guardianship and on how to obtain the legal authority to make decisions on behalf of loved ones.

TRANSPORTATION

In each province, the Ministry of Transportation makes the official decision on when a person with dementia must stop driving. The family physician is *legally* required to report any case in which someone's driving ability may be impaired due to the progression of age or any resulting condition. The physician must file his or her report with a Medical Review Board, which may, based on research and interviews with key health care professionals, request a driving assessment to determine driving skills. Based on test results, a decision will be made on whether the individual will be allowed to continue to drive.

If you are concerned about your parents' ability to drive, you can request an independent assessment for one or both of them. Such assessments, which are provided by private companies for a fee, will help you determine your parents' safety while on the road. Contact the department below for more information.

Newfoundland Department of Works, Services and Transportation
709-729-2300 or 709-729-6997

This department provides driver assessments to determine driving competence.

SPECIAL NEEDS

Canadian Hard of Hearing Association — Newfoundland branch
709-753-3224

The association provides information and brochures on improving communication skills and helping people deal with hearing loss.

Canadian National Institute for the Blind (CNIB) — Newfoundland
709-754-1180 or 1-800-334-2642

The CNIB offers numerous resources including counselling and referral, orientation and mobility training, sight enhancement, and technical aids.

Yukon

TERRITORIAL GOVERNMENT

Home care and long-term care services are accessed throughout the territory by calling the government departments listed below, or 1-800-661-0408.

Extended Health Care Benefits for Seniors
867-667-5403
Range of health services for elderly people who are not covered by private insurance.

First Nations Office
867-667-3399
This office provides home management and personal assistance programs to members of First Nations.

Home Support Program
867-667-5774
This government office will refer callers to numerous home care services such as occupational and physical therapy, as well as nursing and social

work. It also provides home care services such as personal care, support activities, health and safety, and bathing.

Seniors Information Centre
867-668-3383
Funded through Yukon Council on Ageing, the centre provides information on resources. Publishes *Information Please: A Handbook for Yukon Seniors and Elders,* a helpful guide to seniors' services.

GENERAL RESOURCES

Alzheimer Society of British Columbia
(provides services to Yukon Territory residents)
1-800-667-3742
The Alzheimer Society provides educational and support programs to improve awareness and to assist families and individuals coping with the disease, as well as telephone support for families and caregivers throughout the province. Regional representatives, respite managers, and volunteers can be contacted by phone or by visiting a regional resource centre. An information package with more local material and a comprehensive facilities list can be requested at no charge.

Veterans Affairs District Office
1-800-647-1822
Please refer to GENERAL RESOURCES in the Canada-wide listings for services offered.

NURSING AND HOMEMAKING AGENCIES

For nursing and homemaking agencies in your area, please contact the Yukon Home Support Program at 867-667-5774.

HOME HEALTH CARE RETAILERS, HOME SAFETY, AND ENVIRONMENT

A social/intake worker at the territorial home care program will be able to find you the home health care products you require. You'll also find products through the following private companies that operate in your region:

Alpine Health Supplies
867-393-4967

Northern Hospital Supply
867-668-5083

FINANCIAL PLANNING/LEGAL

Office of the Public Administrator
867-667-5366 or 1-800-661-0408
This office is responsible for protecting the financial rights of cognitively challenged people. They help individuals make decisions on personal care and medical treatment. The office also advises family members on guardianship and on how to obtain the legal authority to make decisions on behalf of loved ones.

TRANSPORTATION

In each province and territory, the Ministry of Transportation makes the official decision on when a person must stop driving. Your family physician is *legally* required to report any case in which someone's driving ability may be impaired due to the progression of age or any resulting condition. The physician must file his or her report with a Medical Review Board, which may, based on research and interviews with key health care professionals, request a driving assessment to determine driving competence. Based on test results, a decision will be made on whether the individual will be allowed to continue to drive.

If you are concerned about your parents' ability to drive, you can request an independent assessment for one or both of them. Such assessments, which are provided by private companies for a fee, will help you determine your loved one's safety while on the road.

Yukon Community and Transportation Services
867-667-5811

This department provides driver assessments to determine driving competence.

SPECIAL NEEDS

Canadian Hard of Hearing Association — Yellowknife branch
867-873-6326

The association provides information and brochures on improving communication skills and helping people deal with hearing loss.

Canadian National Institute for the Blind (CNIB) — BC-Yukon Division
604-431-2020

The CNIB offers numerous resources including counselling and referral, orientation and mobility training, sight enhancement, and technical aids.

Northwest Territories

TERRITORIAL GOVERNMENT

For a comprehensive listing of territorial services, go to www.hlthss.gov.
nt.ca

Department of Health and Social Services
867-920-7991
This department provides information on provincial health services and
departments related to home care.

Department of Health and Social Services: Health Promotion Unit
867-873-7371
This government offers support regarding active living, cancer prevention and screening, dental health, and more.

GENERAL RESOURCES

Alzheimer Society of Alberta
(provides services to Northwest Territory residents)
403-250-1303

The Alzheimer Society provides educational and support programs to improve awareness and to assist families and individuals coping with the disease.

Northwest Territories Seniors Information Line
1-800-661-0878
Provides information on home and residential care.

NWT Seniors' Society
867-920-7447
Advocacy for seniors.

Veterans Affairs District Office
1-800-647-1822
Please refer to GENERAL RESOURCES in the Canada-wide listings for services offered.

NURSING AND HOMEMAKING AGENCIES

For nursing and homemaking agencies in your area, please contact the Department of Health and Social Services at 867-920-7991

HOME HEALTH CARE RETAILERS, HOME SAFETY, AND ENVIRONMENT

A social/intake worker at the territorial home care program will be able to find you the home health care products you require. You'll also find products through the following private company:

FINANCIAL PLANNING/LEGAL

Legal Services Board
867-873-7450

This board is responsible for ensuring that all eligible persons in the Northwest Territories receive legal services. The board follows prescribed guidelines for determining if a person is eligible and oversees the operations of legal aid clinics situated in every administrative region of the NWT.

Office of the Public Guardian and Trustee
867-920-5029 or 1-866-535-0423
This office is responsible for protecting the financial rights of cognitively challenged people. They help individuals make decisions on personal care and medical treatment. The office also advises family members on guardianship and on how to obtain the legal authority to make decisions on behalf of parents.

TRANSPORTATION

In each province and territory, the Ministry of Transportation makes the official decision on when a person must stop driving. Your family physician is *legally* required to report any case in which someone's driving ability may be impaired due to the progression of age or any resulting condition. The physician must file his or her report with a Medical Review Board, which may, based on research and interviews with key health care professionals, request a driving assessment to determine driving skills. Based on test results, a decision will be made on whether the individual will be allowed to continue to drive.

If you are concerned about your parents' ability to drive, you can request an independent assessment for one or both of them. Such assessments, which are provided by private companies for a fee, will help you determine your parents' safety while on the road. For a private assessment, please see DriveAble in the TRANSPORTATION section for Alberta.

Northwest Territories Transportation
867-873-7406
This department provides driver assessments to determine driving competence.

SPECIAL NEEDS

Canadian National Institute for the Blind — Northwest Territories
867-873-2647

The CNIB offers numerous resources including counselling and referral, orientation and mobility training, sight enhancement, and technical aids.

Nunavut

TERRITORIAL GOVERNMENT

Services for home care and long-term care are referred throughout the territory from the department listed below:

Nunavut Ministry of Health and Social Services
867-979-7601
This department provides information on provincial health services and departments related to home care and caring for aging parents..

GENERAL RESOURCES

Kitikmeot Inuit Association
1-867-983-2458

Kivallig Inuit Association
1-867-462-4012

Nunavut Social Development Council
1-867-979-6730

Qikiqtani Inuit Association
1-867-979-5301

Alzheimer Society of Alberta
(provides services to Northwest Territory residents)
403-250-1303
The Alzheimer Society provides educational and support programs to improve awareness and to assist families and individuals coping with the disease. The resource centre is open to the public and can provide referrals to support groups in your local area and mail information.

Veterans Affairs District Office
1-800-647-1822
Please refer to GENERAL RESOURCES in the Canada-wide listings for a description of services offered.

NURSING AND HOMEMAKING AGENCIES

For nursing and homemaking agencies in your area, please contact the Nunavut Ministry of Health at 867-979-7601.

HOME HEALTH CARE RETAILERS, HOME SAFETY, AND ENVIRONMENT

A social/intake worker at the territorial Ministry of Health will be able to find you the home health care products you require. Call 867-979-7601.

FINANCIAL PLANNING/LEGAL

Office of the Public Guardian and Trustee
867-975-6334
This office is responsible for protecting the financial rights of cognitively challenged people. They help individuals make decisions on personal

care and medical treatment. The office also advises family members on guardianship and on how to obtain the legal authority to make decisions on behalf of parents.

TRANSPORTATION

In each province and territory, the Ministry of Transportation makes the official decision on when a person must stop driving. Your family physician is *legally* required to report any case in which someone's driving ability may be impaired due to the progression of age or any resulting condition. The physician must file his or her report with a Medical Review Board, which may, based on research and interviews with key health care professionals, request a driving assessment to determine driving skills. Based on test results, a decision will be made on whether the individual will be allowed to continue to drive.

If you are concerned about your parents' ability to drive, you can request an independent assessment for one or both of them. Such assessments, which are provided by private companies for a fee, will help determine your parents' safety while on the road. For an assessment, please see DriveAble in the TRANSPORTATION section for Ontario.

Motor Vehicles Department
867-873-7419
This department provides driver assessments to determine driving competence.

SPECIAL NEEDS

Canadian National Institute for the Blind – Nunavut
403-266-8831
The CNIB offers numerous resources including counselling and referral, orientation and mobility training, sight enhancement, and technical aids.

NOTES

NOTES

NOTES

Notes

NOTES

NOTES

NOTES

NOTES

NOTES